PATIENTS

PATIENTS

by Polly Toynbee

originally published in England as *Hospital*

Harcourt Brace Jovanovich
New York and London

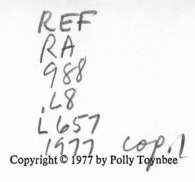

Copyright © 1977 by Polly Toynbee

Printed in the United States of America

Library of Congress Cataloging in Publication Data

Toynbee, Polly, 1946-
    Patients.

    Published by Hutchinson Pub. Group, London under
title: Hospital.
    1. Hospitals—Great Britain.   2. Hospital patients—
Great Britain.   I. Title.
RA986.T68   1977   362.1'1'09421   77-73122
ISBN 0-15-171295-6

First American edition

B C D E

to Tara Walker

Contents

Preface

The London Hospital was a bewildering place at first. It seemed like a puzzling maze of buildings and tunnels, behind its imposing portico which rises above a bleak stretch of the Whitechapel Road in the East End. Heavy traffic rumbles continuously past on the main road out of the city.

The hospital is a jumble of old and new buildings welded together. Many of the surrounding streets at the back have been annexed to it. The private wing, the huge out-patients block, the dentistry department, the medical and nursing schools and many others have grown out into small back alleys and cul-de-sacs. Underground tunnels link some of these blocks to the main building. There is a whole subterranean world running under the hospital, with the shop, the library, the social work department, and dusty gallery after gallery of medical records and old ledgers, all squeezed into these catacombs.

At the back of the hospital a small garden has been almost eaten up by prefabricated dining-rooms. Most of the wards look down on a statue of Queen Alexandra, and a few tall plane trees which add a little grace to the struggling plot of green.

I spent in all five months in the hospital in 1975-6, watching doctors, nurses and patients. The hospital is huge and I saw only a part of it. Even now, when I go back there after visiting so many wards and clinics, I rarely see a familiar face hurrying along the main corridors.

There are 732 beds in the main hospital, and another 1000

in the various other hospitals in the Tower Hamlets area which are now part of The London. The hospital costs over £14¼ million a year to run. It employs approximately 900 nurses, 125 consultants and 300 doctors. It also employs a further 2000 non-medical staff – administrative, clerical, professional, technical, domestic, catering, porters and others.

I chose a teaching hospital and not an ordinary general hospital to write about so as to get a picture of the full range of the National Health, with a few of the top consultants with international reputations as well as the more run of the mill doctors. I chose The London as it is more like a general hospital than any of the other teaching hospitals, as it still has strong roots in the community. The East Enders regard it as their own, and many of them use it as their GP and dentist too. Most of the other teaching hospitals have lost their local roots and rely largely on special or difficult cases being referred to them from outside their area.

Although The London Hospital has agreed to publication of this book, it must be realized that the views expressed are not necessarily upheld by the hospital staff and District Management Team.

Acknowledgements

This book would have been impossible without: Sister Ballisat, Dr Brownjohn, Staff Nurse Anne French, Dr Goodwin, 'Mrs Meg Harris', Alan Hawkes, Professor Huntingford, David Kenny, Dr Kinston, Ros Levenson, Sister Seymour, Dr Silver, Dr Snodgrass, Richard Taylor, Mr Thomas, 'Mr West' and, most of all, Hospital Assistant Secretary Amanda Bass. I am grateful to them all and to the many others at The London Hospital for their great help.

I

Birth

It was eight o'clock in the morning and the ward Sister was coming on duty. She walked along the passage, past the patients' rooms. Most of the women were quietly resting, tired by the effort of getting up. Breakfast and the first rounds were long over.

Marie Celeste is the ante-natal and labour ward. In room after room women in the last stages of pregnancy were lying awkwardly like rows of whales stranded on a beach. The place was quiet, the night staff tired, and all that could be heard was the gentle hum of the floor polishers.

Sister went into the small office at one end of the ward. It housed the computer terminal and a few chairs. She took a clean white apron from a cupboard and pinned it onto her dress. It is the symbol of being on duty. She straightened her tiny elaborate lace cap – a curious garment that looked more appropriate to a waitress than a senior nurse with a large and busy ward under her control.

The Staff Nurse from the night shift came in, eager to hand over and get back to her room to sleep. She carried a Kardex file under her arm with brief notes on each patient's progress during the night. They sat down next to each other and all the nurses on the on-coming shift came in to listen. They each had biros and sometimes jotted down notes on the starched underside of their aprons.

'Mrs Flanigan is being induced today,' the Staff Nurse began, reading out from her notes.

'Has her drip been set up yet?' Sister asked.

'Not yet,' she said looking up with a slight expression of apology. Sister smiled and noted it down first on her list.

'Mrs Allen has been complaining of pains but doesn't seem to be in labour.'

'Well, she's a bit of a complainer, isn't she?' Sister said, and the others agreed with enthusiastic nods.

'Mrs Wheeler's had a migraine. She says she often gets them and I gave her some distalgesic. Mrs Ellery is still getting a lot of pain from those stitches.'

'Yes, I feel sorry for her. They really are very painful indeed.'

'Mrs Catley says she's going to discharge herself today unless we start inducing her this morning, along with Mrs Flanigan.'

'I wish she would, she's nothing but trouble,' Sister said.

'She says she knows she's overdue, but as she's the Professor's patient, I don't think he's going to want to do it, do you? Anyway I doubt if she's overdue at all.'

'Mrs Jones is getting tightenings again and I think they'll have to put her back onto the Salbutamol.' She was expecting twins and needed the drug to prevent premature labour. And so they went on through the list of twenty-three patients.

'No admissions last night?' Sister asked.

'No. A quiet night.'

The Staff Nurse handed over the file to Sister and unpinned her apron. Then she hurried away off duty. The two student nurses went off to their work and the Sister sat there for a moment or two going through the notes alone.

The Sister was a young woman, quiet and gentle. She was a little shy to be a favourite with the patients, though everyone liked her. As she was just getting up to leave the room the telephone rang. The ward clerk, who usually dealt with telephone calls wasn't there so she answered it herself.

'Marie Celeste. Sister speaking,' she said. I could hear a voice, a woman's high-pitched voice, but I couldn't hear the words.

'Yes. All right. Now don't upset yourself,' Sister was saying.

14

'What's your name again? Janet Mercer? Well, you'd better come on in. No, if you're worried get your husband to call an ambulance. He'll bring you by car? Well, you haven't far to come, have you? How frequently are you getting contractions? Not yet? Just the water broken? All right then. You come along in and we'll be expecting you.' She put the telephone back on the hook.

'She sounded in a right state,' she said to herself, shaking her head. 'But she'll probably calm down when she gets in. They usually do.'

She went off to arrange for the setting up of a drip for Mrs Flanigan who was to have her baby induced that day. Mrs Flanigan was a large woman in her mid thirties, but looking much older. This was her first child. On her notes they called her case 'elderly primigranda' which seemed a bit hard for thirty-five. (Primigranda means first pregnancy.) She was in a state of terrible nerves. The other women in the ward were trying to cheer her up. She had been in hospital for well over a month. She had already suffered three miscarriages, and had haemorrhaged once during this pregnancy. 'Oh God, I wish it was over,' she said. Her friends kept telling her not to worry, but there were tears of panic in her eyes.

She was put into the 'first-stage room', where women at the beginning of labour lie and wait. The drip was set up over her bed and taped to her arm. The drug in the bottle was for stimulating the womb to go into labour. It didn't always work. This unnatural labour tended to be quicker but more painful. Mrs Flanigan's blood pressure had gone up, so the doctors had decided to induce, although there was still a month before the baby was due. There was another problem too, one which Mrs Flanigan either hadn't been told, or hadn't chosen to understand. The doctors thought the baby felt too big for its age. It could just have been that she had got her dates wrong, or it could have been what the doctors feared, hydrocephalus – water on the brain, causing the baby to have an enlarged head.

Once she was alone in the room, lying back on the pillows, she seemed to feel less anxious. She tried to sleep for a little, her spiky dyed red hair looking oddly bright against the many pillows.

By this time the corridor of the ward was filling up with young medical students. It was time for the Senior Registrar to take them on a round. This morning it should have been one of the consultant's round of his patients, but he was away, so the Registrar was taking it instead. There were eight students, seven men and one woman. They looked particularly young in their flapping white coats. They had only been on this ward for a week, so their knowledge of obstetrics was small, probably a good deal less than that of most of the patients, some of whom were tremendously well informed with a mixture of obstetric folklore and medical knowledge they had gleaned from keen overhearing in the hospital.

A Staff Nurse sitting at the desk in the middle of the corridor, near where the students were waiting, said quietly under her breath, 'I wish they'd teach them something before they sent them up here to the ward.' But it is the teaching policy of this medical school and of every other one in Britain to teach on the wards, with live patients. This was especially important in obstetrics, where they really needed to see and examine patients to understand what to look for.

There was a flurry down the corridor. The Senior Registrar had arrived. Wherever she went she created an air of hurry. She was a thin energetic woman with hair tied in a tight dark bun.

The students came to nervous attention in her presence. She smiled briefly to them and set off at once to the first room of the ward, the students hard on her heels. She stopped at the end of a bed and the students gathered round as best they could. She talked so softly that those not standing next to her could only hear snatches of what she was saying. The patient could hear it all, and though not included in the proceedings, was not intended to be excluded either. Each of the students had been allocated a few patients on the ward and was expected to be reasonably well acquainted with both patient and case history.

'Whose patient is this?' asked the Senior Registrar as they stood round the bed of one woman, who had been taken by surprise and with a little embarrassment heaved herself up onto her pillows while trying vainly to cover her thighs with her short bright pink nylon nightdress.

One of the students coughed, by way of identifying himself and pushed forward to the bed table where he opened a folder of notes.

'Well, Mr Smythe, would you like to present your patient to us?'

'Um, well,' said Mr Smythe, blushing a little. 'This patient is thirty-four. Her last period was on January sixth. She is gravida. . . .'

'Just a minute, Mr Smythe. So when is she due?'

The student looked hard at the notes but could get no clue from them.

'If her last period was January sixth, when is she due? Well, come on. Don't any of you know? Hasn't anyone told you how to calculate it?'

They said that no one had yet. She raised her eyebrows at them a little, and explained that you add seven days to the date and then nine calendar months. 'So when is this lady due?'

A quick calculation and he said, 'October thirteenth.'

He went on through the notes. 'She is gravida four [fourth pregnancy]. Her first baby had respiratory difficulties. So did her second.'

'Why was that, Mr Smythe?'

'Um, oh yes. They were both premature. So was her third.'

'Yes. That's the most common problem with premature babies, isn't it?'

'Her last baby was breech. She had to have an anaesthetic to remove the placenta.'

The patient at this point interrupted, clearing her throat politely. 'My last wasn't breech. I never had a breech,' she said.

The Senior Registrar and the students looked at her, surprised. 'Well, dear, wasn't it?' she said, brushing back an escaped wisp of hair. 'You know what we mean by breech? Born back-side first?'

'Yes, I know, but it really wasn't.'

'Well, I'm afraid the notes must be wrong,' she said, looking at them again with some puzzlement. 'Never mind.' Then she turned back to the student again.

'So, Mr Smythe, you've told us everything?'

'Yes.'

'Well, then, would you like to tell us what we brought her in for?'

'For bed rest,' he said with some confidence.

'Why should she need bed rest? Have you felt her tummy? Is everything normal with this pregnancy?'

The Registrar bent down and pulled the counterpane over the patient's legs and up to the base of her stomach, and then pulled up her nightgown and began to feel around and press parts of that large stretched-looking mound.

'Come and feel,' she said. The student obeyed. 'That feels like a good-sized baby, doesn't it?' He agreed. 'So why have we brought her in?'

'For bed rest, to stop her having another premature baby.'

'Does bed rest prevent premature labour?'

'Um, yes?' he said uncertainly.

'No. It doesn't. But if she should start going into labour, we have a good chance of stopping it if we catch it very early. If she had come in from home it might be too late to stop it.' She turned to the patient.

'Well dear, I think you can probably go home next week as the baby feels big and we're over the danger period. If anything did happen and the baby was born after that it wouldn't really matter.'

The patient nodded and smiled, and the group moved on to another bed.

'So you can go home then?' asked the girl in the next-door bed in a whisper.

'She said next week,' the patient said gloomily. 'Yesterday

they said I could go tomorrow. You never know where you are with them, do you?'

The Senior Registrar completed her round. She was hard on the students, questioning, probing, not letting them get away with any vagueness of expression that might hide ignorance. She lectured them on the right way to present a case. 'Give the patient's name first, and introduce her to us. Give her age, tell us if she's married, how many children she's had, how many pregnancies, how they ended, whether there were any problems. Tell us how she is and why she's been admitted.' Her round had taken an hour, and she hurried off again to another appointment.

As she left a young couple were coming down the passageway to the ward. The girl was enormously pregnant, wearing a crisp white- and blue-flowered cotton dress. She had long thin legs and looked like a balloon on the end of two sticks. She had glossy long brown hair, and was holding tightly to her husband's arm. He was a little taller than she was, with bright gold hair. He carried a suitcase, an elegant red and silver one. They came to the office at the head of the ward. The ward clerk poked her head out and said, 'Yes?'

'I'm Mrs Mercer, Janet Mercer. I rang,' she said nervously.

'Oh yes, dear, just sit here. I'll fetch Sister.' She bustled away down the corridor. The couple sat down gingerly on the long bench outside the office. He put the suitcase down at his feet.

Sister came down the corridor to meet them. 'Mrs Mercer?' she asked. 'Come along with me, and we'll examine you.' She led her away to the first-stage room, where Mrs Flanigan with her drip was dozing lightly in a bed in one corner. Sister pulled the curtains round a bed in the opposite corner and told Mrs Mercer to get undressed.

Mr Mercer was left alone on the bench. He chatted to the ward clerk rather miserably. 'I went to the class they have for fathers,' he said. 'All the same, you don't feel ready for it when it happens. Will I be able to be with her? I don't know if I can face the last bit.' The ward clerk was a friendly black lady and she laughed and said everything would be fine. She went back to her computer keyboard where she was tapping out the daily bed state – the list of patients in the ward that morning, and their bed numbers.

The midwife who examined Mrs Mercer was a young, athletic-looking Staff Nurse with blonde hair. She would see the patient right through the birth, unless there were complications and a doctor had to be called. She came out of the first-stage room and down the corridor to see Mr Mercer. 'Your wife's fine, Mr Mercer,' she said. 'You can go and sit with her now.'

'How long will it be?' he asked.

'Not for a few hours, I'd say. But we can always be surprised.' He got up and followed her into the room. The curtains had been drawn back and his wife was lying on the high mound of pillows, her long brown hair round her shoulders. She was very pink and pretty. He sat down on a chair by her bed and patted her hand.

'You all right love?' he asked. The chair was low and the bed was high – it emphasized his awkwardness. 'You getting pains?' he asked.

'Just now and then, not too much,' she said. And as she said it she suddenly screwed up her face and clenched her fists. He looked alarmed and took her hand again.

'You all right? You OK?' he asked.

The contraction passed and she said she was. 'It's not too bad,' she said.

'You doing your breathing, like they taught in the classes?' he asked.

'I'll try,' she said.

Sister had asked Mrs Mercer whether she minded my presence at the birth. She said straight away that she didn't. 'Goodness, there'll be crowds there anyhow, won't there, with all the students. What's one more?' she had answered good-naturedly. I was grateful. If I had been her I think I would have refused.

'Now I'm here, I don't feel so scared,' she said. 'When it

started at home, and the waters broke I was terrified.' She began to look around her. She asked in a low voice about the woman on the drip. I told her that her name was Mrs Flanigan and she was having her baby induced because of high blood pressure.

'Oh,' she said surprised. 'Is that all they do to induce it? I thought it was done with nasty instruments.' Her husband winced at the thought. I wondered whether he would be able to watch the birth.

In this hospital every woman in labour is supposed to have someone sitting with them for almost all the time. It is a task left to the medical students and student nurses, under the supervision of a midwife. In the course of their training medical students have to learn the care of women in labour, to witness two births and then assist at fifteen to twenty deliveries. This batch of students who had only just started obstetrics were, for the time being, only expected to observe a delivery. Two of them had been assigned from the morning round to sit with Mrs Mercer and Mrs Flanigan.

The student assigned to Mrs Flanigan was small, mousy and bespectacled. I heard a Staff Nurse briefing him before he went in to sit with her. 'She's lost three babies in the early stages of pregnancy and this time she's haemorrhaged. She has raised blood pressure, and that's why we are inducing.' Then she added, 'This is a precious baby,' which seemed to me an odd phrase to use. The student took the notes and went in to sit with her. He was also given a book in which was a graph to record the progress of labour – frequency of contractions, blood pressure, foetal heart-beat, etc. He had in his pocket a small funnel-like ear-trumpet for listening to the baby through the wall of her stomach. The drip on her arm was to be checked. The patient was to be cheered and calmed.

The student adjusted his spectacles and sat down in the chair beside the bed. Slowly Mrs Flanigan opened her eyes. The student introduced himself, and explained that he was going to sit with her for most of the time. He took her wrist and checked her pulse. He tried to look stern and experienced but then broke into a grin of embarrassment. She gave him half a smile and nodded her head. At the moment the contractions were slight and well spaced.

'You're young for a doctor,' she said, her speech a little slurred from sleep.

'I'm a medical student,' he said.

'Oh,' she answered with a smile, 'One of *those*.'

This unlikely pair were due to sit together for the best part of the day – this mountainous red-faced woman with cropped red hair and sad eyes, and this small freckled student who kept taking off his glasses to clean them on his white coat. What were they to talk about?

'Would you like a drink, perhaps?' he asked, clearing his throat. She smiled and shook her head. There was a long silence.

'Well, it's all going nicely,' he said with false jollity. He knew, and he knew she knew, that he hadn't much more idea how it was going than she had. But she smiled quite kindly. A little later he patted her hand.

'Everything all right?' he asked.

'Yes,' she said. She caught her breath and tensed her face muscles, then the contraction passed. He looked at his watch and noted it down on his graph.

'Well, it's a nice day to have a baby, isn't it?' he said in an avuncular tone that didn't suit his youth.

'Never you mind, son,' she said drowsily. A nurse came in to give her a shot of pethidine, and the boy cleaned his glasses again.

The other medical student, assigned to Mrs Mercer, had a less onerous job. He drifted in and out of the room, and felt no obligation to keep a cheery conversation going. Mrs Mercer had her husband for that. I wondered where Mrs Flanigan's husband was.

Sister asked me along to the nurses' coffee-room. There was a big tin of biscuits on the table sent by a friendly East End trader whose baby had been born in the ward last week. 'Usually all the presents go to the post-natal ward, as that's where they leave from,' said one nurse.

The blonde midwife who was looking after Mrs Mercer came

in. 'How are those two doing? When will they be delivered?' asked Sister.

'Mrs Mercer's fine, but it's going slowly. Not for a few hours yet, I shouldn't think. Doctor's just examined Mrs Flanigan. She doesn't seem to be dilating at all, though she is getting contractions.' She poured herself some coffee. I asked if anyone knew where Mrs Flanigan's husband was.

'I don't know,' said Sister. 'He has been in to see her quite often. But he doesn't even know she's being induced today. I asked her this morning if she wanted to ring him, but she said casually that she thought he'd be too busy to come up today. She says he's self-employed and can't get away from his business. But it is odd, especially as they've been trying so hard for a baby for so long.'

'She told me he'd given up. He didn't want to hope too much this time. He's got superstitious,' said a student nurse.

'There are some mental strains that some people just can't take,' Sister said understandingly.

'I think he ought to. After all, she's got to and he ought to stand by her,' said another nurse, and most of them agreed with her.

After coffee Sister went back to the desk in the middle of the corridor to look through some papers that had accumulated there. Several women in short nightgowns and slippers were crowded round the door of the first-stage room, calling out greetings to Mrs Flanigan. She had been in hospital some time and knew a lot of the other long-term patients well. Some of the women had been in for a large part of their pregnancy.

Mrs Catley was waving to her from the doorway. 'How's it going, love?' she asked, in a loud whisper, perhaps keeping her voice down for Mrs Mercer's benefit.

'Not so good, not so bad,' said Mrs Flanigan.

'Well, it's an effing horrible business, no matter what they tell you,' she said.

'No need to tell me,' said Mrs Flanigan, who felt another

contraction coming on. The medical student turned and frowned at Mrs Catley who withdrew with the others.

Mrs Catley was the woman in the ward who was said to be the trouble-maker. The nurses tolerated her with some determination; she had some nerve, and an irreverent, ribald sense of humour. She was a complainer, not a moaner about herself, but a bossy objector. She complained about the nurses – they weren't polite enough. She complained that the sheets on the beds weren't changed often enough, the food was disgusting, the nurses didn't answer the buzzer fast enough. She was a tough young East Ender about to have her third child. She had a heavy ruddy face and an upturned nose. She advanced towards Sister at the central desk.

'Nurse, aren't they going to start me off this morning?' she asked, in an indignant tone of voice.

'I don't know, Mrs Catley,' Sister answered with a trace of a sigh. 'You'll have to wait for the Professor's rounds. You're his patient and it's for him to decide. I think he'll probably say you must wait.'

'I'll bloody walk out of here if he does!'

'You tell the Professor. Talk to him about it.'

'I will,' she said, gave a sudden surprising grin and shuffled her great stomach back towards the ward.

The students were back in the ward again. It was time for Professor Huntingford's round. Half the patients in the ward were under him, and the other half were divided between the other two consultants. He had then only arrived at the hospital within the last few months, an extremely distinguished obstetrician with much-publicized and outspoken views about the dangers of inducing babies unless absolutely medically essential. But he could not influence the attitudes of the other two consultants. Although he was head of the teaching department, he had no authority at all over the treatment the other consultants gave to their patients.

He was a dark man with streaks of silver in his hair and central European good looks. He had a long list of patients to see, and since he only visited once a week, the patients had built up a measure of hope and expectation for his round. He was the man who would make decisions.

His first patient was in a room on her own. She was a tiny skinny Bangladeshi woman, with a pinched skeletal face and bones protruding. She was known in the hospital as Mrs Bibi. Bibi means 'married woman' in Bengali, a fact well known to the nurses and doctors, but nevertheless ignored for bureaucratic reasons. Her file said Mrs Bibi, the equivalent of being called Mrs Mrs, so she stayed Mrs Mrs, although it was accepted that her husband and children had a different surname. There were often other women patients in the hospital called Mrs Begum, the same thing in. 'They accept it. They know who we mean when we say Mrs Begum or Mrs Bibi,' one of the nurses said.

Mrs Bibi did not speak or understand a word of English. None of the Indian or Pakistani patients in near-by wards had been able to communicate with her as they spoke different languages. She was completely isolated. Her face expressed nothing but despair and misery. She never smiled. Sometimes she would wander down the corridor slowly like a tiny brown ghost and attach herself to a nurse who she would then follow round for a while until the nurse couldn't stand it any longer and took her gently back to her bed where she would sit cross-legged or lie with her thin hand on her brow.

Every mealtime Mrs Bibi was handed out her ration, same as everyone else. And every meal time the food would go cold on her table untouched. She ate only what was brought in to her at lunch time by her eleven-year-old son. Each day he came with a small canister in one hand, trailing his four-year-old brother in the other. He spoke some English but was terrified of the nurses. They tried to get him to translate for them, but these conversations often seemed to worsen the look of doom and despair on Mrs Bibi's face.

The hospital sometimes managed to arrange for translators from amongst the porters or other members of staff, but heads of departments complained at losing their employees at inconvenient times of the day. For real emergencies agency interpreters could be called in within an hour or two but opinions varied as to whether this system really worked or not, and they charged high fees.

'Well,' said Professor Huntingford, with his hands clasped behind his back, when all the students and the Sister had crowded into the small single room. 'We don't know very much about this lady, do we?'

Mrs Bibi lay still on the counterpane with her large hospital-issued vyella dressing-gown flapping round her. Her expression didn't change at all and she looked as if she had no interest in what was going on.

The student assigned to her case thumbed the notes. 'We think she has had four live children and two abortions in Bangladesh, but whenever we ask the family we get a different account. No real idea of dates, but she appears to be very small for the approximate dates given.'

The Professor smiled at her, but got no response. 'Can we feel your tummy?' he asked politely. She offered no resistance. 'Yes, it does feel very small,' he said. One or two of the others had a feel. 'She looks dreadfully undernourished. She needs a lot of feeding up. I think we'd better keep her in, just to be sure she's getting a proper diet. She looks very depressed too, doesn't she? Yes, we'd better keep her in. See she gets plenty of food, and plenty to drink, will you.'

The Professor asked my opinion, and I told him that she ate only the tiny amount of food brought in by her son. 'Is she a vegetarian?' he asked. No one knew. 'Would she eat eggs or cheese or milk? Does she at least get dahl [a nutritious Indian pease pudding]?' But no one knew what she ate. He asked the Sister to see that a dietician was brought in the next time her son came with some food to examine it.

The Professor complained bitterly that although the hospital was in the middle of a large Bangladeshi and Indian community no provision was made for special ethnic diets except Kosher. The hospital records were full of Mrs Bibis and Mrs Begums but there was no translator nor an Indian cook. 'You try to eat more, yes?' said the Professor to Mrs Bibi as he left, but she looked away.

The group moved into one of the four-bedded rooms where a pretty blonde woman was lying. She sat up energetically as they came in.

'How do you feel?' the Professor asked her.

'Fine, fine,' she said with a smile.

'So why have we got you in here, Mrs Maston?' he asked, knowing perfectly well.

She knew, by reputation, the Professor's views, so she answered in a questioning tone, 'To start me off tomorrow?'

'Do you want to be "started off"?' he asked, almost playfully.

'Well, I don't mind, really,' she said, looking at the faces round her for support, clearly giving what she hoped would be an acceptable answer, rather than the truth.

'You have one child already?'

'Yes, she's staying with my mum. My mum's taken two weeks off work, while I have the baby.'

'So it would be very convenient to have it induced tomorrow?' he asked, still twinkling at her.

'Well, you see, now she's arranged for this time off, she can't change it, and she can't take off more time later.'

The Professor turned to his students and said, 'Here is a woman on whom we would be doing an induction for social rather than medical reasons. The baby is quite normal, the mother quite healthy. There is some uncertainty about dates, as she had a somewhat vague menstrual cycle. There is a range of error of at least three weeks. And then you have to take into account that however certain someone says she is about her dates, she could have made a mistake.' He paused and looked at the group. 'What do you think?' No one answered.

'Mrs Maston, it would be a great nuisance, wouldn't it, if we sent you home again? We must take that into account.'

'My mother wouldn't have taken the time off at all if the doctor in out-patients hadn't told me I was going to be started off tomorrow. He said as I was due he'd send me in for induction.'

The Professor sighed, and turning to his students he shook his head a little and said, 'You see it takes a long time to change the policy in a place like this. Those doctors in out-patients are working for me, and under me, but it still hasn't really sunk in with them. I have to tread carefully, so as not to hurt anyone's feelings. They're very anxious to do the right thing and prefer an error of commission rather than omission.'

He picked out one student. 'Well, Mr Oldham, what would you do with this woman? Would you induce?'

The student was about to give the quick and obviously desired answer when the Professor stopped him and said, 'Now don't just tell me what you think I want to hear. I can't bear that,' leaving the young man quite stuck for an answer at all.

The Professor smiled and turned back to Mrs Maston, with a charming manner, 'Now, Mrs Maston, be honest, what do you think? There is no reason at all to induce. We might make a terrible mistake and the baby might be very premature. Is that risk worth taking?'

Mrs Maston gave a reluctant answer. 'I think you're right. But I was started off before, and that was OK. I don't know what it's like not to be started off. It's handy knowing just when it's going to be born.'

'There you are, you see,' the Professor said to his students. 'These ladies have become used to being induced, even though it's usually more painful. They are a bit afraid of spontaneous labour. It's got as bad as that.'

Mrs Maston, having had time to understand how the discussion was going to end, plucked up courage and some indignation. 'Just tell me one thing, Doctor,' she said. 'How is it that one of you doctors can tell me to make arrangements and come in here, and another then say I needn't have come in at all?'

He smiled at her broadly, 'We *are* a terrible crew, Mrs Maston, but I have the privilege of being able to over-rule all the others. It is bad, and I really *do* beg your pardon, but you can go home whenever you like and come back when you've gone into labour all on your own.' He nodded to her by way of indicating that the interview was over, and they all moved on to another patient.

Mrs Maston was a minor victim of the shift in policy at the hospital. She seemed, as she left the ward that afternoon, to feel only a small amount of indignation, but she felt more strongly than ever that she had no hold over her own destiny while she was in hospital. 'They make you feel like a small child, don't they? I don't know why, but it's all this messing you about. So many people saying so many different things to you when they come round each day. You give up trying to make much sense of it all. You're helpless, aren't you?'

The class difference between the doctors and most of the patients was particularly noticeable in the obstetric department, where almost all the women came from the East End, unlike other wards where interesting special cases were brought from all over the country. However hard consultants like Professor Huntingford tried to overcome it, his patients felt they were being patronized, both as lay people not initiated into the mysteries of medicine, and also as poor working-class East End women who had little point of contact with these grand consultants.

The Professor delivered a nasty shock to a young girl in the next bed. He prodded her stomach thoughtfully, pursing his lips and humming and hawing. 'Sister, come and feel,' he said. She did so. He invited two of the students to have a go too. 'Now what do you think?' he asked, rocking back on his heels a little. 'She's anaemic, that's why we brought her in, isn't it? It's a big tummy, wouldn't you say? And I can only feel a rather small baby in there. She's due in the next couple of days though. Any opinions?' He paused for dramatic effect, and no one ventured a suggestion. 'Are we happy about the number of foetuses in this tummy?' The wretched girl looked quite appalled.

'Wouldn't you say that anaemia can often be a sign of multiple pregnancy? And isn't this tummy rather big for the small baby we can feel? I think there may be another one we can't feel lying behind it somewhere. Let's get an X-ray done.'

I asked the Sister what she thought, as we all moved on to another bed. She whispered that she didn't think so. She thought it most unlikely, and, as it happened, she turned out to be right.

The Professor's rounds were over, and Sister sat down at her desk to note a number of decisions he had made and orders he had given. Neither Mrs Mercer nor Mrs Flanigan were his patients. Both had been examined in the meantime by another doctor. 'Mrs Mercer is progressing nicely,' said Sister before I went into the room to see her. 'Mrs Flanigan – not good.'

'Progressing nicely' meant Mrs Mercer was having contractions more violently and more frequently. She looked different, her calm pretty pink cheeks were flushed deeper and her face was tense. She had been given pethidine but was still in pain.

'She's sort of vague,' her husband said, 'And sleepy. But she says the pethidine doesn't make the pain any better. The breathing thing doesn't seem to work. I keep reminding her of it, but it's making her cross so I don't any more. Oh dear, I wish I could help.' He was still sitting on his low chair. He looked lower and smaller in his anxiety. She looked high and elevated on all those pillows and in such pain.

'I know it's silly, but it scares me. I've never been in pain before. I should have been more grateful. Do you think many people suffer this kind of pain much of the time?' she asked. Then she gasped and clutched at the bed clothes. She panted loudly, trying to keep to the breathing exercises she'd been taught.

'She's not *supposed* to breathe like that,' he said anxiously. 'It's called hyper something or other. It's bad for you, too much oxygen.' She relaxed and looked at him wanly.

'It's awful,' she said. 'No one ever said it was really awful, did they; at all those daft classes?'

The smell of lunch came drifting into the room. Two young nurses were pushing a heated metal trolley of food down the passage. One of them poked her head into the room. She withdrew it again rapidly, and said to her friend, 'Oh, they're in labour in there. Are they supposed to eat?'

'Dunno,' said the other. 'It's not like an operation, is it?'

We could all hear them debating and Mrs Mercer called out, 'I don't want any anyway!' which solved their problem and they moved on.

Mrs Flanigan was asleep. The medical student was standing gazing out of the window with his hands in his coat pockets. I asked him how she was. 'They're worried about her,' he said. 'She's not progressing at all, not dilating.'

After lunch had been cleared away and the patients were all resting on their beds before afternoon visiting, Sister called two student nurses over and told them that a private patient was to be admitted that afternoon.

'She's being induced tomorrow morning.' She was one of the consultant's patients.

The Professor, holding a university post, has no private patients, while the other two consultants admit about twenty each year.

Sister said, about private patients, putting it as delicately as she could, 'Well, they vary a lot, but we find there are two types. We don't mind the *really really* private ones. You know what I mean, the ones who are used to money and servants and all that. They behave very well on the whole. But some, you know, they'll press the buzzer for a nurse to come and pour them a glass of orange juice, or turn on the television for them. They ask for things all the time, as if they were staying in a high-class hotel or something. They don't treat us as nurses at all.'

All the nurses found it hard to understand why anyone should want to be a private patient, unless they were foreign and not allowed in on the National Health. It costs £48.50 a day, just for the bed and meals, before paying any medical bills. With ante-natal consultations and ten days in hospital, the average cost of having a baby privately, with no complication, is over £500. The only real privilege is that the consultant promises to deliver the baby himself. (In fact, this particular patient was delivered by a doctor, not the consultant, who happened not to be there.)

The only amenities that the daily £48·50 bought were a pink counterpane instead of a blue one, one meal a day different (but not noticeably) from the other patients', and a telephone.

The other patients could wheel the telephone to their bedside at any time. This ward had a number of single rooms, so that anyone who particularly wanted one stood a good chance of getting one anyway, on the National Health.

It was just after everyone else's lunch when Mrs Bibi's small son was spotted creeping down the corridor towards his mother's room. He was carrying a little tin billy can in one hand, and held his small brother's hand in the other.

Sister saw him and swooped down. 'Can I see what you've brought your mother?' she asked.

The boy looked frightened. He thought he was in trouble. 'Yes, food, for my mother,' he said. He looked smaller than his eleven years.

'Can I see it? What is it?' she asked kindly.

They went into Mrs Bibi's room and he put the canister down on the table. 'What is that food?' Sister asked again.

The boy took off the lid. On the table was Mrs Bibi's untouched corned beef salad, left there from lunch. There was a slice of meat, two slices of tomato, some greyish mashed potato and a few sad lettuce leaves.

'Does she eat meat?' asked Sister.

'No. No meat,' said the boy shaking his head and looking at the floor as if this were a guilty admission.

'Does she eat eggs?'

'No, no eggs.'

'Cheese?'

'No eat cheese.'

'What about milk? She won't drink milk here. Would she drink it if you brought it for her?'

'No like milk.'

'Would she eat fresh vegetables? Look, this tomato,' she said pointing to the slices of tomato on the salad plate.

'Would you tell her she must at least eat her tomato and lettuce?'

Mrs Bibi began talking rapidly to her elder son, while fondling the hair of the younger boy.

'What is she saying?' asked Sister.

'She say she sad. She worry much about small boy when she in here. She want to go home.'

'You tell her the small boy's fine. It's time she started worrying about the one in her tummy. Unless she eats more food there may be a lot to worry about.'

The boy hung his head and did not relay the message. Perhaps he hadn't understood, or perhaps he just didn't like it.

Sister peered into the canister again. 'Is that dahl?' she asked. He shook his head.

'WHAT IS THAT?' she asked finally.

He said something that sounded like, 'Cheep.'

'Chips?' she said with incredulity looking at the brown curry.

'Sheeep,' he corrected firmly.

'Oh, sheep? Mutton? Meat?' she said and he nodded.

'I'm going to get a dietician to look at it next time, you come, all right? It's too late today. You give it to her now,' and she went away, while Mrs Bibi began slowly to eat the tiny quantity of food and rice with a spoon. She pushed away the salad plate with some determination.

It was just a little later in the afternoon that the Senior Registrar examined the two women in the labour ward again. Mrs Mercer's husband retreated rapidly from the room on the arrival of the doctors. The curtains were pulled round the bed and another vaginal examination was performed, to see how far the cervix had dilated to tell how long it would be before the baby was delivered. The contractions were coming more often, and more severely, but though she moaned and tried not to shout, between each one she managed to bring herself back enough to say a few sane and friendly words to her frightened husband.

The doctors retreated behind the curtains round Mrs Flanigan's bed and Mr Mercer crept back to his wife's bedside. A nurse told him that they thought she'd deliver within the hour, and he nodded his head vigorously and swallowed hard.

'Not long now,' he said to her.

She smiled, and said, 'Thank goodness. I couldn't take much more. All I can think of is I want it over. I hardly care what happens. I couldn't care at all about the baby, I just wish it would go away.' He nodded and stroked her hand. Then she was consumed by another contraction and she screwed up her face and panted with the pain. She writhed in the bed, held her breath, then let it out again with the gasp, 'I want to go home! Take me home!'

'You'll be all right, pet, not much longer. You hang on there,' he said, but his voice was shaking with fear and misery. Mrs Mercer's medical student came back in.

'Shouldn't she have some more painkiller? It seems very bad,' the husband asked him.

'Well,' said the student hesitating. 'I'm not sure. She's had quite a bit. Look, I'll go and find out.' He went out of the room to find the Sister or the midwife. While he was gone Mrs Mercer seemed to fall asleep for a few minutes, until abruptly awoken by the next contraction.

Suddenly in the room there was much bustling around Mrs Flanigan's bed. They had decided to put her in a single room for tests – they were worried. The medical student and nurse came rushing out of the curtains round her bed, out of the room and down the corridor. A moment or two later they were back and they helped to drag her bed out of the room, down the passage into a small private room. The Senior Registrar and two other doctors came hurrying along after them; a nurse was holding up the drip still attached to Mrs Flanigan's arm.

In the small room straps were put around her large and mottled stomach. The straps were attached to a machine which was being set up to measure the foetal heart-beat on a screen and a graph. As soon as it was switched on there were loud irregular thumps, the sounds of the baby's heart. Green dots flickered across the screen.

The Senior Registrar was explaining something about her case to another doctor. Mrs Flanigan had had a stitch put into her cervix during pregnancy to prevent her miscarrying again. The stitch had been taken out earlier that day. Thirty-five, she was saying, was old for a first pregnancy. Mrs Flanigan looked a great deal older than her age, perhaps forty-five, I would have guessed.

She was heavily drugged, and apart from an occasional moan, seemed hardly to know where she was. Her head lolled sideways on the pillow. Her face was red. Her hair looked knotty, her hairline sweaty. The Senior Registrar was saying that Mrs Flanigan had made no progress at all in labour. The cervix had scarcely dilated, yet the contractions were strong. There were signs of foetal distress. The baby's heart-beat had gone flat and irregular, and she didn't like the sound of it. She wanted to perform a caesarean quickly, to save the baby from the possible dangers of lack of oxygen if birth were delayed too long.

She telephoned Mrs Flanigan's consultant. The case was discussed by the nurses in the corridors, the students, and the doctors. The patients put their heads out of their rooms to see what was going on, to hear the gossip.

The consultant decided to wait another while before operating. Everyone had another prod at her stomach. Everyone agreed that the baby felt odd. If it was really supposed to be a month premature, then that baby had a very big head indeed. Mrs Flanigan was good-natured, resigned and doped. She didn't mind the prodding, was hardly aware of the air of emergency, and I think managed not to hear any suggestion that there might be something wrong with the baby.

Mrs Catley and another lady were standing in their doorway, almost opposite Mrs Flanigan's single room. 'She never thought it would come right, this baby,' she was saying. 'She always said she just wanted the miscarriage and be done with it. She's had so many go wrong that she's given up hoping a long time ago. If the baby dies I don't think she'll be surprised, not even that sad, poor pet.'

The nurses were divided on what they thought should be done. The doctors felt that if the baby was definitely deformed the woman should not be put through the pain and suffering of a caesarean. It is a nasty operation, with some risk to the mother. It causes great pain afterwards for some time, an ordeal that is almost unbearable if the baby is abnormal or dead. On the other hand, if there was a chance that the baby was all right then it should be saved at once, especially as she was an older woman who might not have another chance. But her previous history of miscarriages made them a little more suspicious about the baby. It seemed likely that it had some congenital malformation.

As they were talking about it the Sister from the ward upstairs, the Intensive Care Baby Unit, came wandering down for a chat with her friend the Sister on this ward. 'I hear you may have one for us soon?' she asked. All babies under five pounds or requiring any special attention are sent to the Unit in incubators.

'I should think so,' said Sister. 'We've got Mrs Flanigan in labour. I think they'll take her up to theatres soon for a caesar, though they've just decided to wait a bit longer to see if she starts making any progress on her own. Feels like a big head though, that's the problem. The Senior Registrar wants to operate right away. The others want to wait.'

'What do you think?'

'I think it is a big head. The baby feels funny. We all think so.' The other Sister nodded and went away upstairs again, to prepare for the possible arrival of another baby. Sister thought that the Senior Registrar would get her way. She told a nurse to get an incubator ready to take up to theatres with Mrs Flanigan as she thought they'd be going soon.

There was still no sign of Mrs Flanigan's husband. Sister asked her again if she could ring him. She didn't like to send her off to theatres without his knowledge. But Mrs Flanigan shook her head. 'Leave him till it's over. He's had enough,' she said blearily.

She was shifted onto an obstetric table to have another test. An amnioscope was used and a sample of the baby's blood taken to see whether it was in distress, whether it was getting enough oxygen. The drip fell out of her arm. A doctor ordered more valium for her.

Then the decision was made. Sister hurried down the corridor to telephone theatres to say that they would be up within five minutes to do an emergency caesarean. Mrs Flanigan was prepared. Suddenly after the delays, the hesitations, the discussions, there was a bustle everywhere. Two porters appeared robed in white. Mrs Flanigan was given a pre-med injection for the operation. A doctor in white wellington boots from the theatre appeared, and the white boots squelched up and down on the shiny floors. People rang other departments on the telephone, orders were issued in all directions. The other patients were watching from their doorways, with excitement and fear. When everything was ready, Mrs Flanigan was hurried down the passage, a nurse running behind carrying the drip. Mrs Flanigan's medical student walked beside her patting her hand as much to ease his anxiety as hers, as they hurried along. A great retinue seemed to follow her progress out of the ward. The midwife in charge of her had hurried away to dress up for the operation and reappeared in the rear in a white gown and hat. The porters trundled along the bed, and then with a rush they were gone, round the corner to the lift and out of sight.

Sister sank into her chair. That was the last the Marie Celeste ward would see of Mrs Flanigan. When she came out of the operation if the baby was alive she would be sent downstairs to the post-natal ward with the other new mothers. If it was a still-birth she would go to a gynaecological ward, away from the sight and thought of babies.

All the drama and excitement was over. The ward suddenly seemed oddly quiet and deserted. Another nurse came and flopped down beside Sister. Mrs Catley came along the corridor, one or two others in her wake. 'How's Mrs Flanigan then?' she demanded. 'She going to be all right? She looked terrible when they took her away.'

Sister answered with a firmness that precluded further questions, even from Mrs Catley. 'She's gone to have a caesarean section. Please go back to your room.' The patients went back muttering to themselves, speculating outrageously.

There was then quiet again, and an atmosphere amongst the nurses of disappointment and thwarted expectation. After all that trouble, all that worry and waiting, suddenly their patient had been snatched away. They were no longer essential participants in the drama, but curious onlookers. They would ring down to the ward later on to see how she was, but only out of curiosity. Their job was over, but they didn't feel they had finished it. They had been cheated of the grand finale.

A little later someone dashed up to Sister. There was a bomb alarm. The big post office on one side of the hospital had received yet another call warning of a planted bomb. Everyone ran round the ward at once. The ward seemed to have filled with more nurses than I had ever seen. Patients' beds were being hauled out of the rooms on one side of the ward into the corridor or into the rooms on the other side. The routine was simple and automatic. It had happened so often before. None of the nurses looked frightened, but they acted with amazing speed.

As the last patients were taken out of the dangerous side a telephone call came to say it was all clear – another hoax. Slowly, and with many jokes and much good humour all the beds were wheeled back again and the walking patients sent back to their rooms.

'It's happened a number of times,' Sister said afterwards.

There have been hoax calls to the hospital itself, but as there have never been specific threats, naming a part of the hospital, patients have never been evacuated because of the danger it obviously involves.

The blonde midwife came up to Sister to say she'd just examined Mrs Mercer. 'She's ready to go into the delivery room now,' she said. Sister nodded and sent another Staff Nurse and a student nurse along to help.

Mrs Mercer's intermittent groans could be heard outside her door. She hadn't been aware of the bomb scare as it had only affected those on the other side of the ward. There was no trouble, no drama about Mrs Mercer's case. Just a routine birth was expected. This young midwife was small and energetic, a little austere and immensely professional.

'You're doing very well, Mrs Mercer,' she said loudly to her patient. 'We're going to take you along to the delivery room now, dear.' Mr Mercer got to his feet shakily. 'Do you want to come?' she asked him.

'Well, yes,' he said. He looked as if he had hoped that at the last minute he would be excluded.

'Just wait here a minute or two, then,' she said.

The two nurses rolled Mrs Mercer's bed out in the corridor and down towards the delivery room. Other patients were watching again. Life in the ward centres around the delivery room. All the women are waiting for their turn to be wheeled in there. It is the holy of holies, the tabernacle from which none of them return, for they are taken straight from there to the post-natal ward downstairs. When someone is in there giving birth, the patients of the ward pass and repass that door. They can hear muffled cries and shouts, loud exhortations from the midwives.

Now already the blonde midwife was shouting to Mrs Mercer, 'Come on! Push! Go on! Don't stop! You're doing well! That's great! Great! Good girl!'

Mrs Mercer had been transferred to the obstetric table, her head and shoulders raised unnaturally high by a mountain of pillows, her legs bent up and spread apart with the great arc light between them. Her husband was standing there by her head, one hand holding onto the table for support, the other sometimes on her brow, sometimes on her cheek. His face was white, his eyes fixed; he never took them off her face, studying every line and movement, lest he should raise them and see anything he couldn't bear.

The midwife sounded like a gym teacher trying to get a fat girl over a horse. She was firm and loud, and I almost expected there to be a referee's whistle between her lips.

The medical student and I were standing as far back as we could get, which was not very far. His face was almost as transfixed as the husband's. This was his first delivery. He tried from time to time to shift his position and to assume something of an air of nonchalance, with little success. I, too, was trying to look calm. Having had a baby myself, and being shortly about to have another, I thought it might be less harrowing for me, but I think I felt it more. I felt it was me I was watching on the table, my baby I was waiting for.

The nurse took one of Mrs Mercer's legs, and the midwife took the other. They rested her feet on their hips so that she could push against them, while they steadied themselves against the bed. As each contraction came the midwife began to shout again. 'Come on! Now! Push! You're not pushing! Mrs Mercer! You're not pushing! Go on!'

Mrs Mercer shouted and then whimpered and moaned, 'I can't, I can't! It's no good, I can't!' Then the contraction would pass and the nurses would relax.

The telephone rang outside in the corridor at the nurses' desk. Sister was sitting there, and she answered it.

One of the nurses from the operating theatre was calling to tell her that Mrs Flanigan was out and being sent down to Mary Northcliffe, the baby was alive and weighed over nine pounds but looked a bit odd. No more news on the state of the baby.

Sister came into the delivery room to give the news to the midwife and nurse. They were pleased. Sister decided to stay and help. Even though she was the senior midwife she became subordinate to the other midwife during the delivery. The midwife in charge remains in charge, and continues to give orders, and make the decisions, so as not to confuse the line of authority, or the patient.

With the next contraction the top of the baby's head became just visible. Mrs Mercer was really yelling, and desperate.

The midwife continued to shout at her, louder this time to try to be heard, 'Come on! You're not trying! It's nearly there! Push harder!' and Mrs Mercer screamed that she couldn't and she wouldn't and it wasn't coming at all. As the contraction passed the baby disappeared and went backwards.

Sometimes the midwife would remember the presence of the medical student and explain to him, over her shoulder, what was happening. Mrs Mercer seemed to hear little that was said to her, except when shouted at very loud. Pain, shock and pethidine seemed to have removed her far away.

At the next contraction the midwife took out a large needle and administered a local anaesthetic to the outside of Mrs Mercer's vagina. 'They don't feel that at all,' she explained to the student. 'During contractions that part is almost numb already.' The baby's head appeared again, a little bigger this time, curiously blue, but again receded with the contraction.

At the next contraction the midwife reached for a pair of scissors and with a loud and terrible snip made an incision to ease the exit of the baby. The medical student and I jumped at the same time. The sound of that snip was far worse than the sight of the blood that flowed from the cut.

Then the midwife eased her fingers in and pulled at the baby. And there, amazingly it was, a big blue head sticking out from between the mother's legs, a bit blood-smeared – but human. There seemed to be such a long, long wait till the next contraction. There was the mother, knees bent up caught in the very moment of giving birth with this extraordinary head protruding from her, suspended in time like a photograph.

Could it have been as long as a minute, or even two minutes, just waiting like that? The baby was so clearly alive already, human, a person, and a person suffering. I panicked – it would die! It couldn't breathe! It wasn't breathing but it twitched its spotty nose and wrinkled its forehead. For all the mother's screams the baby looked as if it was having an even worse time.

The mother was rigid with shock, too astounded even to scream. Then the contractions began again.

41

'Now! The last time! Push, Janet Mercer, push! Push that pain out of you!'

Squeezing her fingers down under its armpits the midwife pulled out the 'pain'. There it lay – on the white table, still blue though rapidly turning pink, the white, yellow and blue umbilical cord thick and shiny in the bright light.

Sister took out a small tube, prised open the baby's lips, while it flailed its fists, and sucked into it to remove any blood or fluid that might have got into its mouth. The baby cried. The mother sighed loudly and painfully: she was still far away and shaking.

'You've got a little girl!' said the midwife. The husband laughed out loud, a squeak and crack in his voice. His wife was still too shocked and exhausted to care, though for a moment she opened her eyes. The medical student dropped his clipboard with a clatter. He had been clutching it too tight and his fingers had gone stiff. His stiff face seemed to crack a little too.

Then, all of a sudden the mother completely recovered. She smiled and the colour flushed back into her pretty pink cheeks – she was radiant. The baby screamed louder and the louder it yelled the more pleased everyone was. It was wrapped up quickly in a shawl, not washed, and given straight to the mother, who was almost too weak to hold it. The father's smile was so wide you could feel it ache with relief. Then she cried and the tears fell from her cheeks to the baby's shawl. Her husband put his head down to rest on hers and for a moment the nurses turned away.

2

Children

The door to the children's ward has its handle set high up where small hands can't reach to escape. Inside the place is always in turmoil, sometimes pandemonium, quite unlike any other ward in the hospital.

A small toffee-coloured boy was heaving the weights off a string at the end of his cot that keep his leg in traction in the air. As he clattered the last one onto the floor, narrowly missing another child building a castle of bricks, he vaulted over the top of the metal bars and tore off down the ward, a young nurse in pursuit.

Opposite his cot, on the other side of the room was a tiny beautiful girl with a thin covering of blonde hair on her baby-shaped head. She looked about five or six months, but was in fact eighteen months old. Her name was Kelly Malloy and she was a favourite with the nurses on that ward – perhaps because she had spent so much of her life there, perhaps because her case was so sad, her future bleak. She sat propped up by pillows, pretty in spite of the obvious oddness of her looks. Her head was tipped back all the time as if the muscles in the back of her neck were too tight. Her head looked big though not too unnatural, and her eyes had a slight squint. They were enormous. She smiled a great deal, and gurgled quietly to herself.

She was born ten weeks premature with hydrocephalus, water on the brain. The London Hospital is well known for its neuro-surgery, so there were many cases of this particular disease in the children's ward, brought from all over the country. The surgeons implanted a tube and shunt – a kind of

43

valve – into the baby's head to drain the fluid that accumulated there. But the shunt often blocks, and sometimes these children have to be operated on again and again to clear it. In her eighteen months of life Kelly had been operated on more than ten times – which was singularly unlucky and unusual.

She had been more or less abandoned by her mother, who was in the process of getting a divorce from the child's father. She rarely visited, occasionaly rang the ward to see how she was. No one knew what would happen to Kelly, but it was generally assumed that she would spend the whole of her life in an institution. She might never walk, and if she did, that would be the limit of her abilities. She was severely brain-damaged.

'She's a dear little thing,' said a nurse, who had stopped by her cot to talk to her for a moment. 'They didn't think she'd live when she was born. Poor little creature, it would be better if she hadn't, I think.' She said that there was no reason for her to be in an acute bed in a hospital, but no one had decided where she would go or what they should do with her. She had fully recovered from her last operation, and was waiting for a decision.

A high proportion of beds in the children's ward are taken up with cases who are there for social more than medical reasons. There are a number of battered and suspected battered children waiting for reports, not really ill.

This hospital has more roots in a community than any of the other London teaching hospitals and in all departments there are many more beds taken up by social cases. Financially, the cost is crippling. Each acute bed costs £300 a week; the waiting lists are long and a wasted bed means more unnecessary waiting for others. The doctors complain of the failure of the social services and the GPs, the lack of local health centres, and of good local hospitals. The social workers complain that doctors still don't properly understand the close inter-relation of health and social needs.

A large number of the hours of a paediatrician's week, both in the out-patients' clinic and in case conferences, are spent on social and not medical problems. Each top doctor at the hospital has an enormous back-up system – the labs, the medical records, the technicians, the administrators, all trying to take the unnecessary work off him, to leave him to practise his expert knowledge on as many patients as possible with the least waste of time. He is waited on hand and foot by the unseen hoards beneath the hospital stairs. It may seem wasteful that he should spend so much time on social work for which he is not trained, yet often that side of his work seemed to be as important, and sometimes more important than the medical side.

Each day in the children's ward there were many doctors' rounds. Most of the children were under the care of the paediatricians first, but were also being treated by the consultants specializing in their particular disease. The neurosurgeons, the orthopaedic surgeons, the cardio-vascular surgeons, and all the others came to see their small patients during the day. The sheer number of people coming and going was bewildering. There were more nurses on this ward than most, and the children themselves tore about and got under people's feet. The illest children were in side wards with glass windows.

There were the parents, mostly mothers but a few fathers, who sat with their children most of the day. They helped to give the place a pleasant air of informality and they chatted to the children with no visitors as well. The nurses recognized that it was vital for the children to have parents there, but sometimes some of the students felt they added to the chaos.

The Senior Registrar was taking a small ward round that morning. At one end of the ward were the babies, then there were the toddlers, and a gate separated them from the older children in the other section.

A high proportion of the babies had bandaged heads and were under the neuro-surgeons, many for hydrocephalus, some for brain tumours. In a corner of the babies' room was a tiny baby girl in a pink suit. She had a huge head and a small body. Her father sat by her all day, often winding up a musical box

45

beside her, but her eyes were shut and she rarely opened them.

In a side ward was a baby boy recovering now from osteo-myelitis of the foot. It had been caused by an infected injection given him at birth in the hospital where he was born. Germs picked up in a hospital can be pernicious, and his had proved resistant to most drugs.

There was another hydrocephalic baby who had his shunt blocked and operated on three times in one week. These valves have to be cleared at once, or the baby suffers great pain.

In another side room an eighteen-month-old girl was in iso-lation. She was sitting in her cot howling behind glass. She had gastro-enteritis, which can spread fast through a ward. Nurses had to wash and gown up every time they went in and out of her room. As a result she got less casual affection from passing nurses and parents, and she screamed a great deal. 'Her mother won't visit,' said the Sister. 'She says she needs the rest. A lot of them say that. They dump their children here and run.'

In the toddlers' section a very active girl was leaping up and down in her cot. She had thin brown arms and legs, and bright curly blonde hair. She bounced all day, and nurses sometimes had to almost tie her down to get her to sleep. She was three years old, and had bruises on her face: suspected battering. They stopped to discuss her case. The houseman was there too, a woman. She said, 'We've got some photographs we took when she came in. You can see definite finger marks on her face and on her backside. You couldn't get a clearer case.' The Registrar examined the pictures, and saw that the bruises took the shape of a human hand.

'She's very lively and friendly,' said the nurse. 'Her mother brought her in herself. She must have been worried. The child wasn't ill, just bruised. I don't know if she was worried about herself or someone else attacking the child again. She hasn't been in since, or phoned. She may be scared.' The little girl reached out for the doctor's notes and then grinned and bounced again. He chucked her under the chin and tickled her fingers.

Then there was a baby in an oxygen tent, a heart case, and next to it a very white baby with a bald head with curious markings on it in indelible purple ink. It was undergoing deep X-ray treatment for a brain tumour. The marks were to direct the machine to the same spot on the head each day. The baby was having a general anaesthetic every day for the treatment, as there is no other way to keep small children still enough.

They stopped by another small child. The nurse said she was having trouble giving her eight injections a day. She had run out of places on her poor punctured legs. 'There just isn't room for eight a day, her legs are so tiny,' she complained.

The Registrar agreed to stop some of them. 'It's too cruel,' he said with a sigh. 'How did we ever get up to eight?' They all agreed that the prognosis for this baby was very bad.

Many of the older children were much less severely ill than the babies. There were more routine appendectomies, fractures, circumcisions, children under observation after falls or taking poison. In one corner was a boy of eleven yelling at the top of his voice, swearing and screaming. He had a leg in plaster hung from the ceiling. A big X-ray machine had been wheeled in beside his bed, a small Pakistani lady radiographer was attempting to X-ray his leg. 'Fuck off! No, no,' he shouted. 'I won't! Bugger off out of it! I won't! Leave off! Leave me alone!'

His mother was with him, a tiny shrivelled East End woman with a shocking orange jumper and holes in her tights. She was embarrassed and apologetic. 'Come on, Gary, just take a minute,' she was saying feebly, looking round at the nurses. She clearly had no control over him.

'You fuck off too!' the boy turned on her. 'You fuck off out of it with the rest of them fuckers! I ain't letting no one, no one!'

The radiographer was losing her temper. 'You silly boy, it doesn't hurt. What will all the others think of you, making a fuss like a baby?' she said.

'I don't give a bugger's fuck!' he yelled, this time with a sob in his voice, angrily wiping away tears.

A Staff Nurse came up and tried an authoritative tone. 'Gary, do as you're told!' But she got nowhere either. The doctors on their round paused to watch for a moment. The mother caught the Registrar's elbow and whispered loudly. She explained the boy was upset because the radiographer was a Pakistani. The Registrar told the nurse to leave it for the moment. He could have the X-ray another time when he'd calmed down.

'I fucking won't,' sobbed the boy.

There was a ten-year-old black girl called Princess who tailed the nurses all day long. She would slide her hand into one of theirs and follow them wherever they went. They were kind and patient. Although she was plain and fat with oddly scaling skin, they often took her on their knee and hugged her. She had a brain tumour.

We walked back down the ward again towards the babies. Kelly Malloy was still sitting there. A nurse was playing with her and she chortled. The doctors stopped by her cot. 'She does seem to get a little better, doesn't she?' the houseman said to the Sister.

'Oh, since she's been in here this time you wouldn't know she was the same child. She likes it here. I don't think they ever bother to talk or play with her at home,' she answered.

'Has her mother been at all?' the Registrar asked.

'Not for two weeks. She hasn't phoned either.'

'What will happen to her?' the houseman asked.

'There's a case conference about her this afternoon,' he groaned. 'Nothing will be decided of course. It never is.'

It was the end of his round and they went back to the Intensive Care Baby Unit where they spent most of their time. I stayed and talked to the Sister.

'People think that all nurses love working with children,' she said. 'But it's very difficult to get paediatric nurses. Most of the nurses don't like paediatric work. It's much harder, and much more chaotic. Some of them say it upsets them too much, but most of them just can't take the noise and the muddle in the ward.'

Everywhere else in the hospital patients are kept in order. Individualism is not encouraged. The patient learns rapidly that to be popular he must be patient, moderately jolly, and not get in anyone's way. Most conform rapidly to this norm on arrival. I met plenty of patients who confided, 'I'm not really myself in here. I'm just trying to fall in with the others.' The one or two people in a ward who are unwilling or unable to conform quickly feel the powerful disapproval not only of the staff but of the other patients too, who have rapidly adopted the hospital expectations of patient behaviour.

Anyone who makes even moderate extra demands on the nurses is regarded as getting in their way, and thus depriving the others in some way. As in totalitarian states, the greater good of all may turn out to be the greater good of none.

But children are exempt from all these pressures. They can scream, complain, spit out nasty food, refuse to do what they are told, and are under no obligation to be grateful to nurses and doctors. Gratitude is expected from anyone over fourteen and under eighty. The nurses and doctors would hate to think that they expect gratitude. They are unsentimental about their work and for the most part will discuss their work and their careers in just the same way as anyone else – in terms of satisfaction, reward, promotion, conditions and excitement. They do the job because they like it, and they would not admit to expecting gratitude from their patients. But that expectation is always there, in one form or another. It is part of the patient–doctor relationship. The older patients brought up before the National Health are quite overcome sometimes by the 'goodness' of the nurses and doctors. This tradition is quite as strong in most other patients. Those who regard their treatment as a right are disliked, reasonably enough, since most people demanding rights are in a self-righteous and aggressive state of mind. But somewhere the balance of gratitude and right has tipped in the wrong direction. It may be sheer terror of the power of doctors that makes patients apologetic and grateful.

In the children's ward the nurses have to deal with a lot of their patients through an intermediary, a parent, who is not a patient, and has to be treated as something of an equal. The student nurses, who are not children-trained, complain sometimes of the 'clutter of people' but I think what upsets them is the uncertain line of authority.

Miraculous work is done in the Intensive Care Baby Unit. Tiny scraps of life are nurtured in incubators into normal healthy babies. Any baby weighing less than five pounds is sent here at birth. Most of the babies here, though, had been born elsewhere and transferred to this highly specialized unit from far and wide, with a collection of rare and serious ailments. Every day battles for life were won and lost here.

The Registrar showed me round: little scrawny flower-pot-coloured arms and legs, tiny bandaged heads, some under the helmet-like breathing masks of respirators – so much machinery for such pathetically small creatures.

Several of the babies I saw were almost certainly badly brain-damaged. I asked the Registrar if they really fought as hard for them as for the others. He said hesitantly that he thought they did. It was impossible to know how many seriously handicapped children lived as a result of their treatment. 'You never know quite whether they would have died without it,' he said. But then added slowly, 'I think, if you want to put it in those terms, that for the sake of the one or two who surprise us, who live and grow up to be quite normal against all the odds, we have to fight for them all.' I asked how he could make a decision like that without knowing how many handicapped children they were making live for the sake of the exceptional case who completely recovered.

'Well,' he said painfully, 'perhaps it would be better if some of them died, But who are we to decide?' He admitted that if he was head of the department his policy might be a little different, but not very much so. 'Those decisions rarely arise to be made, I'm glad to say.'

Dr Snodgrass, a young man and dynamic paediatrician is jointly in charge of the unit. He is an expert in inborn metabolic disorders and much research is carried out under him in this department. Babies born with an inability to metabolize certain proteins and other substances are sent here from far afield.

'Dr Snodgrass believes that initially they should all be resuscitated,' the young Registrar said. 'There is one baby here who has been on a respirator since he was born, three months ago. As far as we know he has no brain at all, not enough even to keep the heart and lungs functioning on their own. His EEG is now quite blank, one straight line. There seems to be nothing there. The parents come often to see him, and they just sit and look at him. They don't know what to think about it.'

Dr Snodgrass came to join us while we were talking and he listened. Then he said, 'The thing is you can never, never be certain. There are no hard and fast rules about any of these things. Babies on respirators with apparently nothing going for them at all have suddenly recovered and grown up into normal children. Take the example of a twelve-year-old boy I once had here. He fell into a canal and was absolutely undeniably observed to have been under the water for half an hour. He was taken out dead. It took half an hour for the ambulance to get here, and there seemed to me no doubt at all that he was dead. There was just no sign of life. But we put him on a respirator and six weeks later he walked out of here with an IQ of 110. How can I ever be sure after something like that?'

But the miracles are relatively few and far between. I felt it was a terrible sadness for parents to lose a new baby, but in the long run, I felt it was a worse sadness to let them live severely damaged in the vain hope of a one in a hundred miracle.

'I don't accept that at all,' Dr Snodgrass said. 'It's not our fault that they were born that way in the first place, and we have no idea which ones would have died on their own and which ones would have survived anyway.'

It so happened that later in the week, with the parents' approval, the doctors decided to take the baby with no brain off the respirator. The baby then frightened them all. It stopped breathing at once, but an hour later it suddenly started to breathe again. Then it stopped for another hour, to all intents and purposes dead, but it started again for a very short while.

Finally it did die, but no one could have said when exactly – or whether it had ever been alive.

The telephone rang on the desk, and at the same moment the Registrar's bleep in his pocket went. An emergency case was on its way, a small four-month-old from Woking with liver failure. They conferred for a moment. Very rare for liver to fail at that age, it usually happens at birth or later on. It was almost certainly a rare metabolic disorder, perhaps tyrosinosis. The baby was unconscious, almost dead. The Registrar hurried downstairs to wait for the arrival of the ambulance.

Dr Kinston was a psychiatrist particularly concerned with trying to help mothers whose babies had to be put into intensive care at birth. He believed that they had serious trouble relating normally to their babies now and in later life. Each week he held a small conference with the staff of the two maternity wards and the staff of the Intensive Care Baby Unit. He was partly lecturing the nurses on their duties to these mothers.

'All pregnant women fear for the health of their unborn baby,' he said. 'As much as there is the wish for the ideal baby, so there is concern at producing a deformed foetus. The delivery of a premature baby comes as a particular shock. Because of the precipitate labour the possibility of a damaged baby becomes a reality. The mother is now in a real predicament: on the one hand she wishes for recovery to take place, and, on the other, she has to deal with the possibility of her baby dying. That she feels responsible for the baby's state creates guilt which is painful. Some mothers find it very difficult to deal with the discrepancy between their image of the baby and the tiny infant in front of them.'

'When babies come up here to the unit they don't look human inside all this machinery. It is very hard for the mother to respond. Animal studies show the danger of separating a mother from its young, even for the first few hours after birth. The mother doesn't recognize the baby as her own and the maternal feelings don't come through. We are very concerned that the mothers should make as much contact as possible with their babies here; to look and to touch, even if it only means holding a small hand through the incubator. There was a study at Stanford University that showed that mothers who had had minimal early contact with their low-birthweight babies had very real problems in relating to their children after discharge from hospital and there were subsequent marital difficulties for the parents.'

It happened that one of the cases that was being discussed that day was one I knew a little about from the maternity ward. The case was that of Mrs Flanigan, the woman who had got half way through labour but had to be given a caesarean at the last moment.

'I find this a most disturbing position for the mother to be in,' said Dr Kinston. 'She has had four very nasty miscarriages and she came to believe that it might not be possible to have children. Her husband was desperate for a child, especially a son, and she longed for one too, but what's happened now is that she seems unable to come up here to the ward in spite of her strong hopes for the baby. It is very worrying.'

A nurse from the maternity ward said, 'We had all that trouble about the baby being abnormal before it was born. I didn't think she'd taken it in, but perhaps she did. Perhaps she still thinks there's something the matter with it.' This nurse had helped care for Mrs Flanigan when she was in labour. 'Do you remember we all thought it had a big head when we felt it? Some of the doctors didn't want to do a caesarean on her because they thought the baby felt so odd.'

'It didn't half look odd too, when it was born,' said the jolly Sister from the Baby Unit. 'We stared at it, and one of the doctors said it had a something or other syndrome, very rare. Its head was a funny shape and its neck was too short. We thought it looked so odd. But then the father came in to look at it, and we all burst out laughing. It looked *exactly* like him. There was no doubt about it. He was a funny-looking fellow, and his son was just a replica. There's nothing the matter with the baby at all!'

'We had to drag her up here to see the baby. I know her

53

stitches hurt from the operation, but after a few days we had to force her. She just sat there vaguely looking at it. She didn't seem to want to know,' said a nurse.

'It does seem odd behaviour,' said Dr Kinston.

Then a young nurse who had been silent until then suddenly said to him angrily, 'You're a man. How do you know what's odd? That woman went through terrible labour for a long time and then had to be rushed to theatres. It's a bloody painful operation and the stitches really hurt for a long time. All we did was to try and drag her up here to see something ill. I think I can sympathize.'

'All the same,' said one of the Sisters, 'she's better now. It's been a long time. At first she'd do anything rather than come up here. She sent her husband if she could.'

'It's taken her six years to have a child and she doesn't know what to do,' said the doctor. 'When did the baby go down to her in the ward?'

'Yesterday. We've been observing her,' said the post-natal ward Sister. 'I think it's just her character, not anything especially to worry about. She's just very vague and dopey anyway.'

'That's true,' said the ante-natal ward Sister. 'She's been in the ward for a good few months so we all know her very well. She's rather a delightful vague sort of person, nice, but not all there. I think maybe she's a bit dim and she doesn't ever think anything is important. She's not very responsible. I get the impression her husband rules her completely, and she just does what he says, and he does a lot for her. She didn't seem all that anxious in the ward. She wasn't that upset at the thought of losing the baby. She thought she would, and she just thought "what a bore" a lot of the time. Everyone liked her.'

'She didn't want to go up to see the baby. She just said to me, "When are they sending it down",' said a nurse.

'That's not always a bad thing,' said the post-natal Sister. 'The ones who go on and on pestering to have their babies every minute of the day are often the ones who don't care so much when it arrives. We can't tell anything yet until she's had total care of the baby for a few days. She hasn't done any feeding or changing it yet.'

'Well, we'll just watch her carefully for the next four or five days then,' said Dr Kinston, and they agreed to discuss Mrs Flanigan again before she went out of the hospital.

A little later in the day there was a case conference on Kelly Malloy, the pretty little girl sitting propped up in the ward. The conference took place in Dr Snodgrass's out-patients' clinic.

There was a long list of people who were supposed to attend, summoned by the paediatric social worker – but almost invariably, some crucial person failed to attend. This time it was the Malloy family's social worker from Tower Hamlets where they lived. However, the senior social worker, the missing man's boss, was there. So were Dr Snodgrass and his Registrar, the Sister from the children's ward, Kelly's physiotherapist and a student nurse.

They all waited a long time for the missing social worker, then finally the paediatric social worker gave up and decided to start without him. She handed out a roneoed summary of the many previous case conferences that had been held on Kelly.

Kelly was born ten weeks premature at a near-by hospital and transferred to The London at two days. She was a tiny baby and her prognosis at birth was poor. She stayed in hospital for six months, having many operations on the shunt that had been inserted for hydrocephalus. She caught several minor infections on the ward. Her mother didn't want Kelly home, was terrified of her. She had an older daughter, Michelle. The mother said that the father used to beat her up. He said he only beat her up because she went out at night, leaving the children alone. She blames him for Kelly's state as she says he kicked her when she was pregnant and that brought on the birth prematurely. No one knew if this was true. The child was admitted again several times for a blocked shunt. This last time she had been admitted three months ago, had been operated on twice, and was now well. Then the mother said she didn't want her back at the moment though she hadn't said she wouldn't take her ever. The father wanted her, to take her to live with his parents. Kelly's mother said she'd take her rather than let her parents-in-law have her.

A summary of the ward Sister's report was read out. She said there was little evidence of the mother showing much care for the child. On her few visits she spent her time discussing her own problems with the other mothers and paid no attention to Kelly. She had to be asked to change the child. Kelly made enormous advances since being admitted to hospital. She responded to all the stimulation given by nurses. Mrs Malloy had not been in contact at all in the last few weeks.

The paediatric social worker gave her own report. She was clearly against the mother and in favour of the paternal grandparents. 'Mrs Malloy expressed aggressive feelings in connection with the social work offered her in the past by the hospital. She stated that she did not like the previous social worker because "she did nothing to help me". But the records show that the social worker concerned spent a great deal of time with the Malloys in an endeavour to sort out their various problems, not least their removal to a more salubrious area.' The Malloys lived in a near-slum on a run-down Victorian council estate. The social worker then went on to say that she liked the look of Mr Malloy and his parents, who often visited Kelly. They were keen to have her and promised that they would bring her to the hospital for physiotherapy three times a week.

There was then a written report from the missing social worker, who clearly had more sympathy with Mrs Malloy. 'Conditions in the home were found to be good. The apparent rejection of the child by the mother was because Mrs Malloy was terrified of abnormality in any way. Mrs Malloy has been seen in the vicinity of the hospital but says she does not come in for fear of the embarrassment she would suffer if she met her husband, whom she is divorcing, or her mother-in-law. She now has a coloured man-friend, and this is not a relationship to be discouraged.'

The paediatric social worker who was chairing the meeting said then that the father was under suspended sentence for beating up the mother. 'But he's never been done for violence before and says this was just because she neglected the children,' she added in defence of him.

The ward Sister backed her up. 'The few times she's been into the ward she's refused to bath, feed or change Kelly. She always comes with a boy-friend, and there have been lots of different ones.'

'Yes,' said Dr Snodgrass, 'I remember she's always had peripatetic habits.'

The paediatric social worker said, 'She keeps giving different reasons why she won't visit. First she's afraid of meeting her in-laws and her husband. Second she says Kelly always cries when she leaves so she feels it's better not to come at all. Third, she says she's afraid Kelly will die, and she can't bear it.'

'Nonsense!' said Dr Snodgrass. 'We've been over it often with her. She knows quite well that Kelly isn't going to die. That was only at the very beginning. Who's she living with? I mean is it some psycho who doesn't like kids, especially handicapped ones?'

The paediatric social worker said, 'I wish the case worker was here as she has a good impression of Mrs Malloy.' There was no one there to speak up for the mother, and no one who knew what the mother thought and felt, or what she really wanted for the child.

'But what about the woman's love life?' Dr Snodgrass pursued.

'I'm afraid I just don't know, except what I've read you from the case worker's report,' she answered.

'I'm not asking for the gory details,' said Dr Snodgrass. 'But when the mother's out who looks after the children?'

The social worker answered, 'She says a neighbour listens through the walls.'

'Aaaah!' said Dr Snodgrass with a disgusted gasp echoed by the others. He felt they weren't getting anywhere. 'The father says he wants to arrange for his parents to take Kelly. Who knows anything about them?'

Here the social worker began to put their case. 'The father is only violent with his wife. He presents as an effeminate sort of man. He's gentle with Kelly on the ward. His mother says she'll give up her job and look after Kelly.'

'But she's never looked after Kelly before?' asked Dr Snodgrass.

'But she does visit almost every day,' she answered.

'That doesn't prove they'd be capable of managing on their own. Kelly is quite a responsibility. How old is the husband?'

'Seventy-five,' said the social worker.

'Good heavens! That's not very suitable,' said Dr Snodgrass.

Sister said, 'I don't think Mrs Malloy would let Kelly go to the in-laws.'

'I'm a bit nervous that, if we suggest it, Mrs Malloy might just come and take Kelly away one of these days, and we couldn't do a thing to stop it,' said Dr Snodgrass. 'She needs careful watching. But I doubt whether those grandparents have the slightest idea what looking after the child involves. Oh, she's a sweet enough little baby now, but what about later? I think we should put her in a foster home for the moment. We can see how highly motivated those grandparents are to get her out of there.'

Sister said, 'I don't think the grandparents know at all how handicapped she'll be. They aren't very bright. They aren't capable of visualizing what it would be like even if we spelled it out to them. Will she ever walk do you think?'

The physiotherapist said, 'Yes, I think she might, if we can only keep the physiotherapy going. I know if she goes into a home no one will bother to bring her. They never have time. I've had that happen often before.'

'What about finding a foster home then?' Dr Snodgrass said.

'It's quite unrealistic to even consider it,' said the Tower Hamlets supervisor. 'We'll never find anyone.'

'So it looks like a home for the moment? Mrs Malloy would accept that? Of course we can't actually decide until we've had more reports from the case worker who knows the family. We'll leave the grandparents as a possibility, but it really doesn't sound to me as if that will be at all suitable,' said Dr Snodgrass.

Then he had to go to another appointment. He apologized and left. The discussion continued for a little while, and everyone agreed to wait a little longer for the case worker to report. People got up and began to leave.

'They really fought for her life,' said the Sister. 'It's sad, isn't it.'

The social worker said that once Kelly had gone into a home she couldn't see her ever coming out again.

Dr Snodgrass was holding a paediatric clinic over in the out-patients building that afternoon. The first child was one of his triumphs, one of the ones that made it all, for him, worthwhile, one of the ones who, against the odds, came through when people like me would have wanted him to give up.

Ruby was a year and a half old, black and very active from the moment her mother brought her into the room. She opened drawers, reached for things off the desk, and wriggled off her mother's knee the moment she was put on it.

Dr Snodgrass listened to her heart, and examined her. He asked her mother what she could do. Did she talk? 'Yes, quite a lot of words.' She had had hyaline membrane disease, a heart murmur, pulmonary haemorrhages, was born at twenty-six weeks' gestation (the norm being forty weeks) and had weighed under two pounds. She had been on a respirator and the brain waves registered not much hope for her. But all the same, here she was, absolutely normal, as far as Dr Snodgrass could make out.

The next child was a healthy little boy of six, Johnny, who also had a heart murmur. Dr Snodgrass listened and said that as was usual in such cases in children, it had cleared itself up, and his heart was now as good as anyone else's.

As he left the room with his mother and small brother, a terrible noise could be heard outside in the corridor. It was a wild, demented, enraged shrieking, and it hardly seemed to stop to draw breath. The orderly came in with some files.

'What's that?' asked the doctor.

'A princess, a devil, a real spoilt one, if you ask me. I know what I'd give her,' the clinic orderly said, shaking with indignation and frustration. She was an elderly orderly with white hair and a comfortable round body inside her uniform. 'I really don't know what it's coming to. And her mother not doing anything to stop her. You know why she's screaming? She wants to pull down all the pictures in the passage and tear them up. She's already had two of them!' She whisked out of the room again; the noise reaching a crescendo every time the door opened and closed.

The next patient was a tiny boy, aged three. He was accompanied by his mother and grandmother. All three of them suffered from the same very rare hereditary condition, quite incurable and unpleasant to look at. They had almost no hair, dead-white very flaky skin, no eyelashes, and tiny pink eyes, no finger nails. The mother was illegitimate, and so was her son. She hadn't wanted the child, but left it too late for an abortion.

The GP's letter said the mother was in a bad way, extremely anxious and nervous, and the child, as a result of his disorder was suffering great pain on defecation, one of the symptoms of the syndrome. His eyes too were inflamed – he had no tear ducts.

Dr Snodgrass talked to the two women while the child wandered around the room picking up bricks off the floor. He tried to comfort them a little, but they were a lonely and desolate trio. There was not much he could do, he said, as he had said to them before on the many other visits. But he'd see if the eye specialist could do something about the child's eyes.

As they got up to go, again the dreadful noise could be heard outside.

The nurse came in, her hands cupping her ears, and announced that there was a representative from a drug company sitting outside. Would he see him? Dr Snodgrass said he would.

A smooth young man, or at least a young man rather rough

at the edges, but trying hard to be smooth, came in, with a slight glance over his shoulder, as if glad to get into the haven of the quiet room from the storm in the corridor where he had been waiting.

He turned on his representative's manner, shot out a hand, and shook Dr Snodgrass's very vigorously. He began his patter, with a fixed beam on his face. He was young, didn't know anything about medicine, but had learned how to sell, or so he thought.

'You'll find it's very good for epileptics,' he said, as he displayed an obscenely glossy folder of brochures about a drug he was peddling. 'In clinical trials eighty per cent of fits were stopped. Very good too for hyper-activity and destructiveness. Also you can't overdose on it. In Australia a man took one hundred times the prescribed amount with no ill effects whatsoever. . . . It really is a marvellous drug. . . .'

Dr Snodgrass was surprisingly polite and gentle with the man, until he started trying to sell an antiseptic cream. Then he cut him short and said he wouldn't use it in paediatrics.

'Very good for nappy rash,' the man persisted.

'No, we wouldn't use it,' Dr Snodgrass said.

'They use it in West Ham football club, you know,' said the huckster. 'It's a wonder for bruises, dispels blood clots under the skin.' Finally, reaching the end of his patter with another beam and vigorous handshake, the man went.

'Straight out of the school for meaningless talk and gestures,' said Dr Snodgrass with a sigh. 'Why do I agree to see such people? Well, it's one of the big drug houses. I do use one of the drugs he was talking about. I like to know what's around, I suppose. No, I don't suppose someone like that would influence my prescribing habits at all.'

The noise, the wailing and screaming outside hadn't abated for one moment.

The next child was brought in, Tracy Brewster. A very young mother and father accompanied this four-year-old girl.

'She's been suffering abdominal pain, you say?' Dr Snodgrass asked, examining the GP's letter.

'Well, she had it a bit in February and March, and then again when she had a tummy upset in October,' her mother said anxiously.

The doctor asked if that was all, and the parents said yes, it was. He examined the child, and asked where it hurt, when it hurt. 'All over,' the mother said.

'I know what you're thinking,' Dr Snodgrass said, when he had stopped prodding the girl's stomach. 'You think it's something called a grumbling appendix, don't you?' The parents looked uneasy, as if they didn't like to admit it.

'Well, I'll put your mind at rest. There is no such thing, and there never has been. A lot of people get abdominal pain, and then of course some of those get appendicitis at some stage, but the two things aren't connected. You've either got appendicitis, and you know it, or you haven't. There's nothing in between.' He then explained to them that a great many children suffer some abdominal pain, for no particular reason. 'It's like grown-ups getting head-aches and back-aches. It's the way they express worry, I suppose, but it's really nothing to fuss about.'

They went away quite happy. I asked why he had been consulted about something so utterly trivial as slight stomach-ache many months ago. It was the sort of thing most parents would hesitate to trouble their GPs with, let alone a consultant.

'Well, there's nothing I can do about that. If the GP service were better it wouldn't happen. But even then, if you get fussy people like these parents, they may have pestered the life out of their poor GP until he sent them to me in desperation. Most of the consultants spend a fair amount of time on cases that should never have been referred. I once had a scribbled referral note that even said, "Temperature?" with a question mark! Because the GP hadn't even bothered to take it himself.'

A very silent girl came in next, with a small baby on her knee.

'Who did you see last time you came?' he asked her.

She couldn't remember. She seemed almost catatonically silent.

'The baby looks fine,' he said encouragingly.

'I get these terrible headaches,' the mother said at last.

'Would you like to see someone about that?' he asked.

She said she would.

'How is your eldest? How is her stammer?' he asked again.

'Just the same, maybe better.'

'Look, I'll put down on your card for you to have an appointment to see the psychiatrist about those headaches. You always know you can come back and see me any time you like.'

She thanked him, and went away, unsmiling and silent.

'I'm very worried about her ability to cope with children.' Dr Snodgrass said after she had gone. 'She's very disturbed. She won't ever admit it, but I'm sure she's been in and out of psychiatric care before. She always says she can't remember who she's seen or where she's been.'

At last, it had to come, it was the turn of the child who was making all the noise. The nurse led in a tired fraught-looking dark-haired woman, dragging after her a screaming howling girl of five, rather fat, with a wet swollen face, contorted with anger not misery. She was kicking with her legs, and clawing with her hands, and the noise was louder and more unremitting than anything I had ever heard come out of a human being.

The noise was so great that the interview had to be conducted by shouting and repeating. The girl kicked her mother in the shins, tore at her clothes, pushed her off the chair. The mother moved to another chair and the girl pushed her off that one too, so she went back to the first. She kept this up through the whole session.

The mother was Greek and she spoke good English but with a strong accent. 'She's been having these screaming fits day and night, day and night for a long, long time. I can't go on. I can't do anything.' The child pushed her off the chair again and thrashed her with her arms. The mother went on talking while trying to ward off the blows. 'What is it with the child?' she asked.

'How long has she had these fits?' he asked.

'Three months and two weeks exactly. I can tell you because it all started on the day she saw her father electrocuted. He was fixing the refrigerator plug in our flat, or so he say, and he put his finger in it and he fell straight off the ladder dead on the floor. She was standing in the doorway and she saw it happen.' There was something curiously casual about the way she told the story, as if it hadn't been something that had also happened to her. 'They say it was an accident. I know he killed himself. He always wanted to kill himself.'

The screaming went on. The child began to reach up for her mother's hair to drag on it and clutch at it in handfuls. The nurse put her head round the door, to see if there was anything she could do. Dr Snodgrass waved her away.

'How often does this happen?' he asked.

'Sometimes only two or three days a week, but once it starts it lasts all day. She can't stop. I want to shut my ears, shut the door, get away.'

'What she needs is a child psychiatrist, not me,' he said. 'I'm going to refer you to someone else in the hospital and mark it urgent. This just can't go on, can it? I can't understand how you've managed at all, all this time.'

The woman took out her handkerchief and burst into tears. 'If you knew my life! I am beaten all the time, everything is dreadful! I have eight children and we live in one tiny flat. They won't re-house us. We owe rent. My eldest has gone to live with his fiancée. The others stay home and fight all day. We all hate that flat. The children are all frightened to go into the kitchen where the accident happened to my husband. They say it's haunted.'

'Are your other children all right?' he asked. The little girl had gone round behind her mother and was beating her back. The screaming hadn't stopped for one moment. I didn't know it was possible to keep up such a noise for so long without pausing to draw breath. The tears still poured down her small cheeks.

'The other children? They are out of control. The eldest one hits me all the time. They all keep climbing up the fire escape at the back of the flat because the lift is out of order always. They go up to the roof and I can't stop them. Those stairs are dangerous. We only have two bedrooms for all of us. Now this screaming is driving them all mad, and they get worse because of it. They can't stand it and they tell me to shut her up, but I can't.'

Dr Snodgrass was leaning across the desk, his face transfixed with horror. It was the only time I saw him looking really appalled by any case.

'Your problems need sorting out, and quickly,' he said.

'Ah, I've had a tough time,' she said drying her eyes and putting away her handkerchief. 'I'm on tablets for my nerves but they don't help.' She sniffed. 'If I could only get re-housed, everything would come right. If I could get her away from that flat she might get better.'

'I'm going to try my very best,' he said. The conversation was still being carried out at the tops of their voices.

He wrote something down on a card and a piece of paper. 'Take that to the Sister. I've told her that it's urgent. You must bring the child back to the psychiatrist this week, you understand? We can't have you live through this for another week, can we?'

She got to her feet and shook him very warmly by the hand. 'Things will get better for you. Don't worry. We'll get things going. If you ever feel you're not getting what you want, or if for any reason you need help, just come back and see me any time, won't you?' he said, as he shook her hand.

Then there was the problem of how to get the girl out of the room. She was lying on the floor kicking with her heels. Her mother pulled her up and she lashed out. The girl bit her arm, but the mother didn't flinch. The girl was more or less dragged out of the room, and we could hear her progress down the network of corridors for some time. Dr Snodgrass sank back into his chair and put his hand to his brow. 'My God,' he said and drew a long breath. He looked quite shocked. 'My God,' he said again.

The orderly came in with some notes for another patient. 'Ooh, what a right one she was. I'd tan her backside for her, I would, the little actress,' she said tut-tutting as she bustled out again.

'I suppose,' said Dr Snodgrass composing himself, 'that the family must be known already to every social worker in the area. They couldn't have fallen through the net, not with a problem that size. I expect she's been in and out of some kind of psychiatric care herself. Did you notice how odd her behaviour was? She had completely cut herself off from that child. She didn't notice it at all. She said the noise got her down, but to take it for three months! No, there's certainly something odd and removed about her. That little girl was battering for attention and the more she tried for it the less she got.'

He was speculating about the child and the social services. Inside the hospital he had complete control over everything and everyone. His writ ran – but the moment he had to deal with anyone outside it was a matter of going down on his hands and knees and begging. The doctors often find the Tower Hamlets Housing Department difficult to influence, and the doctors try to restrain themselves from writing too often about too many of their cases. Sometimes they pick up the telephone and try talking to them about the very worst cases – the tiny babies sent home to wet basements, the cardiac cases on the top floors of tower blocks where the lifts fail. Sometimes it works, sometimes it doesn't. The Authority, say the doctors, have their own priority cases and priority list. Any amount of money seems to be on hand inside the hospital to have a patient wheeled around by porters, escorted, cosseted, but once he's outside the door, and the chill wind is blowing down the Whitechapel Road, he's on his own, and there's nothing much the doctor can order for him there.

Health and Social Security are lumped together, but often it's hard to see where they meet. The social services of the borough are now co-ordinated so that the hospital social workers belong to the same team, and are paid by the borough.

But that's a small administrative matter. The real difference between Health and Social Security is money. The amount of money spent on bringing hospital treatment up to the level of such luxury and care is remarkable, when compared with the poverty of many of the patients' lives.

Was there ever a time when anyone looked at our priorities and decided that it was all right if people lived in squalor, undernourished, ignorant and helpless – but if they got too bad and developed an acute ailment they should be taken away and given the very best of whatever was available to cure that particular bit of them, and then send them back to where they were before? Is it done in the name of making sure that we all have the same right to life, even if it means that less is done about the quality of some people's lives?

If you ask the doctors at the hospital questions like, 'How many houses could you build for the money spent on intensive care, keeping alive poor handicapped children, or wretched patients on kidney machines? How many people could you prevent from ever getting ill in the first place with the money you spend on treating one patient?' they give the very reasonable but fatalistic answer: 'If the hospitals spent less and cut back, what makes you think the government would spend it on housing and preventative medicine?'

Perhaps there is some hope of change of attitude to medicine and preventative medicine. Recently the Department of Health and Social Security brought out a pamphlet called *Prevention and Health: Everybody's Business*. It makes the point powerfully that in the past the great breakthroughs in health have had little to do with medicine, but more to do with the building of sewers and drains and houses. The doctors accept that historical fact, yet it looks as if it will be a long time before anyone understands its full implications.

Seven o'clock in the evening, a final ward round was in progress. Some of the children were asleep. The naughty brown boy who kept throwing the weights off his leg in traction was still doing it, three or four times an hour. He would tear down to the older children's part of the ward, just reach the door with the high handle before some nurse would catch him and plant him back into his cot.

The little battered blonde girl was still bouncing up and down – thump, thump went the springs of her cot. She guffawed with glee when anyone came near her. In another bed nearby was a small black boy, lying inert gazing at the ceiling. He had been stabbed, but was not seriously ill.

The father was still sitting by the baby in the pink suit, winding up her musical box for her automatically, although her eyes were closed. Nearby a nurse was feeding a small baby. The baby in the oxygen tent was back in the open air, and smiling.

The older children were watching television. The boy who swore at the radiographer was roaring with laughter at some silent joke relayed through his head phones. A girl recovering from an appendectomy was finishing a game of Monopoly with a girl with a septic foot. Kelly Malloy was lying curled up in her cot, a sleeping cherub, her gold curls a little damp on the pillow, her thumb in her mouth.

'She'll be going soon,' said a nurse who was tending a restless child in the next bed. 'We'll miss her.'

3

Patient

It was an ordinary Thursday morning in a busy clinic, one of
the busiest, the general surgical. The consultant was away and
his Senior Registrar, Paul Thomas, was conducting it. I was
there to select a patient to follow all the way through his or her
hospital stay, and because choosing one was so difficult, I had
decided to take the first person who was about to be admitted
within the reasonably near future.

There were three jovial-looking medical students there, one
man and two girls. I sat next to them, and whispered to the one
nearest, 'Is there any particular speciality this morning?' He
smiled and whispered back, 'Oh no, just the usual, lumps and
bumps and things, mostly.' Medical students rarely fail in
their chilling jocularity. Is it insensitivity from lack of experience? Or gaucheness, making light of what still shocks them
greatly, but doing it with excruciating clumsiness? Or just a
youthful desire to shock? I don't know, but I smiled back.

Mr Paul Thomas gave a severe nod in my direction before
reaching for the first sheaf of case notes on his desk. He was a
dark, heavy-set man. Although young, probably in his mid-
thirties, he had an aura of authority that stopped the medical
students' whispers with half a glance. The room was tall, with
high ventilators leading out to the street; half sentences wafted
in oddly from time to time. The press of people waiting outside the door were quite silent. Why are patients so patient?
Why are they prepared to sit outside doors in dingy corridors,
clutching their appointment cards for mythical appointments,
long past, with hardly a murmur of complaint? They have

become lumps of meat, patients, and they have discarded already their outside identities. They are 'lumps and bumps', hernias and gastric ulcers, not housewives, grocers, welders or clerks.

The first few patients were regulars, returning after operations for check-ups. Mr Thomas tossed a set of notes to each of the students and told them to go and examine a patient each in one of the nearby examination rooms. They were to see the new patients, and take a lengthy case history from them, write methodical and legible notes to read back to Mr Thomas before he examined them himself.

The ginger-bearded student departed with the case of Mrs Harris under his arm. The two girls left the room with their patients. While they were gone the doctor got through two routine cases. He said that hernias and breast lumps were much the commonest.

The students spent a long time with their cases, and it was half an hour before the bearded one returned. Mr Thomas swung round in his chair. 'Well?' he prompted somewhat brusquely. The young man cleared his throat nervously. The students were only in their second week with this 'firm' (a group of doctors under one consultant).

'Mrs Harris is forty-six, married with two children. Two weeks ago she noticed a lump on her right breast. On examination she has a large craggy lump on the breast. It does not appear to be attached to the skin or muscle. I can't find any indication of other swellings. . . . Family history – she has a sister who had a breast removed twenty-five years ago and who is alive and well. She breast-fed both her children. Her younger son has cardio-vascular disease and is awaiting surgery.' He showed a diagram he had sketched of her breast, showing the exact position of the lump, and also showing one or two shaded areas where there were slight hardnesses.

Mr Thomas nodded and asked one or two supplementary questions, more to test the student's knowledge than to ascertain important information about the case.

'Well, let's go and see her,' he said rising from his chair. The student led the way down the corridor past the staring faces to a small cubicle of a room, and I followed on behind.

They agreed that it sounded almost certain that the woman had cancer. For my benefit the doctor explained that at that age a large and 'craggy' lump almost invariably meant the worst. If the student's first examination was right, there was a reasonable chance that it had not spread yet, although it was a large lump. The fact that it was not attached was a good sign. The doctor spoke in a serious straightforward way. He dealt with any number of these cases all the time, but he was not in the least off-hand or callous. He was grave and un-dramatic.

The room was like a sleeping-car compartment on a train, except with no window. There was just room for the couch and standing room for three or four. We squeezed in.

A woman was lying on the examination couch, one arm up behind her head, the other lying across her naked breasts. She was of medium build, with dark, tightly curled hair. Her body and face were bronzed from the recent heat-wave sun, except for her breasts, which were bright white and full, and round. She was a handsome woman; her face was only a little lined. The contrast between her tanned face and her white young-looking breasts with their taut skin and bright raspberry nipples gave me the odd sensation of looking at someone with their head stuck through one of those cardboard models seaside photographers use; the head and body didn't seem to belong to one another. Nudity often gives that effect.

She looked up as we came in, and there were tears forming in her eyes. She tried to wipe them away quickly before anyone saw, but since we were all squashed together so very close to her, she hadn't a chance of hiding it. She sniffed, tried to smile and said a little hoarsely, 'You mustn't mind me. I'll be all right in just a moment. It's just that all this couldn't have come at a worse time.'

The doctor gave a faint smile, the student beamed with embarrassment and I looked at my shoes. The doctor continued to fix her with his firm eye. I think he was trying hard to look friendly and honest, but not to give her any false hopes which might have to be crushed. He wanted her to know that he could be trusted and that he would tell her the truth. He didn't go in for the 'well, well, what-have-we-here?' avuncular cosiness of some doctors.

The woman looked up into his face, tried to smile, but her lips quivered and the tears began to fall, down her cheeks one or two onto her bare breasts, and the student and I left the room.

The doctor came back to his consulting room quite soon, leaving the woman in tears to be helped to get dressed by a nurse. 'Yes,' he said. 'We'll have to admit her on Monday for operating on Tuesday.' I asked how sure he was that she had cancer, and he said, 'Well, one always hopes, and I might be wrong, but I'm pretty certain. Though you never can tell until you see what's there.'

Quite soon she was shown into the room by the nurse, and she was now composed, and managing to smile. The doctor rose from his chair as she sat down. 'Your husband's outside isn't he, Mrs Harris? Would you like him to come in too, or would you rather not?'

'Oh, please ask him in,' she said with a look of great relief on her face. 'I haven't any secrets from him, you know. He's so good. He always goes everywhere with me.'

The door opened and the nurse ushered in Mr Harris, a tall good-looking man also newly bronzed from the sun. He was carrying a small suitcase which he put down under his chair discreetly.

'Well, Mr Harris,' said Dr Thomas, 'I've told your wife that I'm afraid she will have to come in to have that lump removed as soon as possible. If it is what we all fear she will have to have her breast removed, but we can't tell at this stage. It's a question of what we find. I say this so that you know where we stand.' The husband nodded, his wife looked towards him to see how he reacted.

'How soon can you do it?' Mr Harris asked. 'I've brought her things in case you want her to stay in today.'

'I've put her on the list for coming in on Monday. That's soon enough.'

'Yes, doctor,' said Mr Harris. His wife, who was feeling much more relaxed after crying, began to talk.

'I'm sorry to have taken it so bad, doctor, but it really couldn't have come at a worse time. My youngest boy, he's eleven, he's waiting for heart surgery. He has a bad heart, from the time when he had tonsillitis five years ago. It was a one in a thousand chance but it went to his heart and we've been waiting to hear when they'd operate. My oldest starts his O Levels on Monday, and it'll be terrible not being there. Well, my sister had the operation years ago, and she's all right, so it's not that I'm especially afraid or anything, but what a time it's come at!'

'Was it rheumatic fever that your son had?' the doctor asked.

'No, the doctors said it was just tonsillitis,' Mr Harris said.

'Is there anything else you'd like to ask?' Mr Thomas asked.

They said they didn't think so, but then Mrs Harris asked, 'How long will I have to stay in?'

'Well, that depends,' he answered. 'If we just removed the lump it'll be about a week, but if we have to go ahead it'll be two or three weeks.'

He had a habit of fixing patients with his eye, so as not to seem to be hiding anything. The Harrises looked a little abashed and afraid of him.

As they spoke he had been filling out her admission forms.

'We'll see you on Monday then, eleven o'clock. You'll be in Sophia Ward. Take these forms to the TCI desk. When you arrive on Monday go to the Admissions first of all. Good-bye.' They rose to go, and were effusive in their thanks. The doctor was brief, and perhaps a little embarrassed by their warmth and gratitude.

The nurse led them away and directed them to the TCI desk. TCI sounds technical and complicated like much that goes on in hospitals but turned out to mean only 'To Come In'. No doubt patients puzzle over the significance of those initials as being somehow relative to their case, perhaps containing the vital clue to the exact nature of their ailment. Terminal Cancer I? Total Collapse Imminent? Hospitals don't realize how much significance is poured into every small phrase.

The Harrises made their nervous way through the procedures. Afterwards she said, 'I was numb when I left that room. I didn't know where I was going or what I was doing. Thank God I had Bob there to get me through all the formalities. Of course I knew really that this was just what would happen when I went in there, but you always hope, don't you? I thought the doctor just might say, "Oh, that's nothing, just a slight spot, or a boil or something." But I knew he wouldn't, didn't I?'

The next Monday was hot, though the hospital was mercifully cool. Eleven o'clock is usually a peak time for the Admissions Office, but by chance it was empty when I came in, except for a reception clerk in front of her computer keyboard, silently tapping away. The computer is still a novelty at the hospital, and is used in all the wards for the bed state, waiting lists, and admissions. Each morning ward clerks have to do the bed state, tapping out the names and bed numbers of all patients. She wore a pink overall, like all administration staff, clerks in admissions, ward clerks, medical records clerks.

I waited and Mrs Harris still didn't come. I wondered whether she had lost her nerve. Fifteen per cent of patients default at the last moment, sometimes even urgent cases like hers.

Then she came in, with her husband behind her carrying her small suitcase. They looked nervous, but not terrified. I wasn't sure how she would greet me. Mr Thomas had asked her before whether she would mind my following her stay in hospital and she had said at once that she would be delighted – 'It'll be something to take my mind off myself!' she'd said kindly. Perhaps when it came to it she would have changed her mind. She was going through one of the most terrible times of her life, and I would have understood if she had decided she didn't want me there after all.

But when she saw me she hurried over and sat down beside me. 'Oh, I'm so glad you're here!' she said. 'A friendly face, someone I know – that really makes me feel better.' And then I felt better too.

The clerk called us over to the desk, and we sat down. The clerk was quiet and matter of fact – not especially friendly. She was so busy dealing with the forms and the computer that she didn't seem to have time to make a special effort at setting Mrs Harris and her husband at ease.

'Are you Mrs Harris?' she asked. She said she was. 'That's odd. I've got your name down on the computer, and your age is given as seventy-six. You're obviously not seventy-six.' The Harrises laughed and said she wasn't.

'Could I have your correct date of birth?' asked the clerk.

'February 20th, 1929,' she answered.

'Your full christian names?'

'Margaret Gladys Harris.'

'Maiden name?'

'Morely.'

'Occupation?'

'Well, I haven't really got one. I used to be a telephonist.'

'Shall I put housewife?' asked the clerk and Mrs Harris nodded.

'You are married?' She nodded. 'Husband's occupation?'

'Transport foreman.'

'Children?' She said she had two.

'Religion?'

'Oh, well, we aren't really. C of E, I suppose.'

'C of E, then.'

The clerk went on writing while we sat in silence. Mr Harris whispered something to his wife and she smiled.

'Well,' said the clerk. 'You'll be in Sophia Ward. A lady will come and show you up there in a minute, if you'll just wait over there for a little while.'

'Can my husband come with me?' she asked. The clerk nodded and pointed to the row of chairs. We got up and went over to them.

'Do you think it matters we were a bit late? She didn't say anything about it,' Mrs Harris said. I said I didn't think it mattered. 'You see,' she went on to explain, 'I wanted to go past the school where my little boy is so I could wave to him in the playground. They come out at eleven and I told him we'd stop and wave.' Had the children been worried? 'My little one didn't seem to be, he was very good about it. The older one stopped his ears and refused to listen. He didn't want to know.'

Another woman in a pink overall came out of a room and approached us. 'Are you Mrs Harris?' she asked with a large smile. 'I've come to take you up to the ward. Will you follow me?'

We got up and followed the woman down the long main corridor. The building is old, but the inside of the ground floor has been done over in an attempt to make the place look new, with bright wood-panelled walls. The strip of carpet down the middle makes the place seem warmer and a little less institutional.

I don't know if our guide ever did any other job, but she appeared to be a professional chatterer, an official putter-at-ease, a sort of hospital Red Coat. Her patter was limited but its range led us exactly to the door of the ward. 'Isn't it warm today? Have you come far? It's such a nice ward you're going into, I'm sure you'll like it. Have you been in here before? Oh, you've never been in hospital before, except to have babies? Well, well, now you'll be able to see how it compares to *General Hospital* and *Angels* on the telly, won't you? They say the weather's going to break soon, but I don't see much sign of it. Don't these lifts take a shocking time to come? I expect you'll be glad to get in the ward and put your feet up, after coming all that way this morning! Here we are, I'll just pop in and tell Sister you're here, just wait here on this bench, dear.'

She left us on a long bench outside the ward on the second floor, and disappeared. 'Didn't she *talk*,' said Mr Harris, and we all laughed with relief. The talk had made us all tense. It had been as if she was trying to think of jolly things to say while leading someone to the scaffold.

'I didn't tell the boys I had to come in until yesterday evening,' said Mrs Harris, 'Though I'm sure they must have guessed, I kept saying to Ian, he's the eleven-year-old, "You know where your socks are," and, "I've put all your clean shirts and pants in the top drawer." So he must have thought, but he didn't say anything. When I told him he said, "Don't worry Mum, we'll manage fine. You just get yourself better quickly and don't worry about us." He's so good like that, isn't he, Bob? He's so considerate to me all the time, so grown up. He's a wonder. The older one, Tom, he hides his feelings.'

I asked if they knew what she'd come in for. 'Not really. They think it's something in my insides. Though maybe Tom knows. He doesn't say much but he has sharp ears.' We waited quietly. 'By the way, do call me Meg,' she said. After that we were on christian-name terms. I asked if she'd like me to go, if she'd rather sit with Bob on her own. 'Oh no, for goodness' sake don't go!' she said. 'I feel you know your way around a bit, you know what we're supposed to do, I feel so lost. I feel like the first day at a new school. I don't feel like a grown-up person here.' So I stayed, for the first time at the hospital feeling I was actually some use, rather than just extra work for everyone.

A nurse came out of the ward. 'Mrs Harris? Will you come with me? We'll just get you undressed and pop you into bed. Would you wait here, Mr Harris. I'll call you when she's ready.' She led her away. I wasn't sure why her husband wasn't allowed to go too. She would have preferred to have him there, she said later. But hospital segregation of the sexes was absolute. If a woman was undressing, no man should be present. Husbands didn't count any more. She was another female patient, entering the discipline of a female ward, and she was not allowed to undress and get into bed with her husband present. It was part of the ritual, and it reminded me of a curious and unpleasant tribal wedding ceremony. Hospitals are good at denying the reality of any life for their patients outside the institution. Your outside identity falls away as you become a patient. Away she went, the nurse taking her suitcase, and we were left to wait. She looked back at us for a moment, and was gone.

'I feel terrible,' Bob said, a little later.

I couldn't think what to say to make him feel better. I longed to say, 'I'm sure it'll be all right. Don't worry. It's bound to turn out to be something quite harmless, just a cyst.' But I knew that Mr Thomas was pretty certain of his diagnosis. All I could say was, 'Well, it's the waiting that's worst. At least you'll know soon.'

'We do everything together, Meg and me. We're very close, never go anywhere on our own. What would I do?' He stopped, and then said, 'Well, she only just noticed it so it can't have gone very far if it is cancer.' I said that catching it in time was what mattered.

'Do you think they'll operate today?' I said no, it would be tomorrow.

'That'll just be the first small one. I wonder how soon they'll do the next one, if she has to have it done?'

I said I didn't know.

'I'd do anything in the whole world for her, you know, Polly,' he said. 'I'd sell everything and get it done private. I wouldn't mind if I spent the rest of my life paying it back. Would it be better to have gone private? I did think I would, except they took her in here so soon. Would she get better doctors?' To have been able to work and pay would have made him feel so much better. The helplessness of sitting and waiting and contributing nothing made him feel bad.

I said that for something serious, there was nowhere better than a big teaching hospital. The only reason for going private was to be in a private room, to get better hotel conditions, but not better medical treatment. Otherwise, for something that was an emergency, where the National Health would admit someone at once, as they had admitted Meg, there was nothing to be gained. She had already jumped the waiting list, so it would just be a waste of money. I explained that the best specialists in Harley Street were the same people who were consultants in the best hospitals, like this one. You paid your money to see the same man, get the same treatment, but in nicer surroundings. He was a little comforted but still not quite believing. 'I thought the rich always got better medical treatment?' I said that for minor ailments, they did. They didn't have to wait three years to have their varicose veins out, or to have a painful arthritic hip or knee replaced. But when it came to the big operations, you could pay out a fortune, and, perhaps, in a small private clinic get worse nursing care, even if you got better food. The rich don't queue, and don't mix with the hoi polloi, but they don't live longer.

Bob Harris was no radical. He voted Labour, but was not much of a socialist. He just assumed, passively, that everything in life was unfair. Although he seemed to believe what I said, he would still rather have been able to pay, and to imagine that he could help his wife. Getting it all free didn't suit him.

'It seems to me,' he said, 'that the things that are most important in life, health and the kids' school are things I'd like to pay for. But they are the things we're stopped from paying. I'd feel better if I could.'

Some twenty minutes later the nurse returned. 'You can come now, Mr Harris,' she said. He got to his feet and went off into the ward to see her, while I waited.

The three medical students went past, and waved gaily at me. I waved back. One of them stopped. 'She gone in then?' I said she had. 'Does she seem like a good one to you?' I said she seemed like a very good one, rather stiffly. By this time I had identified with the Harrises so much that I disliked the feeling that I might get any confidences behind their backs, that doctors might tell me anything about her. I wanted to keep them all at a distance. I didn't want to know what they thought of her.

Soon Bob came out and beckoned to me to come and see Meg. I went after him into the ward, down a long passage with two rows of beds on the right, and into a long brighter room at the end where two rows of beds faced each other.

Meg had gone into the ward carrying her neat navy coat over one arm. Her brown mock crocodile shoes with a gold buckle had made a crisp clacking on the floor. Then she had disappeared inside the curtains round her bed. She had been shown her locker, told to unpack and undress. All her possessions had been closeted away in the cupboard. Her shoes went away and instead her slippers were tucked under her bed. All the clothes that belonged to the outside world were hidden away – and when the curtains were pulled back as I approached, Meg Harris had turned into the patient in number ten bed.

She was sitting in her slot, in a crisp white flowered nightgown and a small bed jacket. She looked so like the others at first glance that I didn't spot her at once when I came into the room. But there she was – transformed into a patient.

'I do feel funny,' she said. 'Why am I in bed? I'm not tired or ill.'

I didn't know why she was in bed, I suppose for convenience, keeping everyone in their slot, so you know where they are. They don't take up so much space lying down. She was wearing a name-tag on her wrist, Margaret Gladys Harris and a long number. She glanced at it and said, 'Well, I'm glad they won't think I'm the wrong person in the operating theatre. Though Harris is a common name. I'd rather have a funny name just now.'

Bob looked awkward standing by the bed. He felt lost, as if he didn't have anything to do with her any more, as if she'd been taken away from him. He smiled sheepishly. Hospital visiting is dreadfully unsatisfactory, and the closer the relationship the more excruciating the occasion. She smiled at him bravely and held his hand tight. 'You'd better go now, love. You'll be very late.'

'Never mind my being late!' he said with surprising vehemence. She laughed, squeezed his hand and said, 'All the same, I think you should.'

A nurse came up. 'I'm afraid you've missed your lunch, Mrs Harris. We have it at twelve o'clock here. I could probably find you a salad and a pudding though, if you're hungry.'

'No, thank you, dear, I couldn't' said Mrs Harris.

'Not just a pudding then? There's some nice semolina and

jam?' said the nurse. Mrs Harris refused, politely. When the nurse had gone she said, 'I want to keep off the hospital food as long as I can. I had a good breakfast.'

She turned to Bob who was especially embarrassed in the presence of nurses. 'Go on, off with you!' she said. He kissed her and left, promising to be back that evening. Meg almost had a tear in her eye but turned to me. 'I'm glad I've got you here to talk to. It takes my mind off things,' she said.

It takes a determined recluse to avoid knowing everything about everyone in a short time in a ward. But I was surprised how much Meg had got to know about many of the other patients in the short time it had taken to get into bed. She explained quietly to me, 'This old lady next to me on my left, she's a dear sweet thing, in terrible pain with leg ulcers and a stomach ulcer. I was chatting away to her, but she's stone deaf, can't hear a thing. Her mind's all there – she reads all day, but she can't hear. She smiles at everyone though. This one on my right though, she's lovely. She's had her breast off, just a week ago, but she looks as fit as anything – and ever so cheerful. I can't understand it. She doesn't seem a bit upset. She's a dear, looks after a lot of the others, goes about cheering people up. How does she do it?'

I looked across discreetly. The woman was in her early sixties, with short fairish dyed hair, glasses and a smiling face. She was sitting at a table close by doing a jigsaw with two other women.

'She's older of course, and she's not married, so perhaps she doesn't mind so much,' Meg said doubtfully. 'I can't stand to think about it. You know I had a bath yesterday evening, and I wore my bra, because I was afraid to look in case the lump had got any bigger. I didn't want to see. I just lay there in that bath staring at myself, thinking, "This is it, I won't look like this again. I'll say good-bye to my breast."' She was quiet for a moment and I couldn't think of anything helpful to say, so I just listened. 'It may sound silly but I've always been proud of them, my breasts. They're very good ones. When I was young, me and my girl-friend used to wear really tight shirts. I remember once going out with her on our bicycles and meeting a couple of boys. It's always stuck in my mind. We got chatting and I heard my one say to the other, "I'm lucky, I've got the one with the best boobs!" and I was really pleased, because I know they are nice. Do you think I'm daft talking like this? But, they're still nice, although I've breast-fed two children. They didn't go small and flabby like some people's. . . . You know my older son, Tom, well he's at that age now, sixteen, where he sits about with his friends, and I hear them making jokes about my boobs. I pretend not to notice, but sometimes he says things like, "Mum, run and get me this or that," and I know he just wants to see me running, to see them wobble.' She poured herself out some orange juice from the top of the bedside table. 'After they've taken out the lump, I wonder how many days it is before they go ahead and take the whole thing off, if they have to?' I didn't know but said I thought it would be soon afterwards.

I left her for half an hour to go down to the canteen to get myself some lunch. The Sister told me, as I passed her desk, that the doctor would be visiting Mrs Harris in half an hour's time.

When I came back through the ward a young houseman was there, standing by the Sister's desk. He introduced himself. He was a stiff and sombre young man, serious and unrelaxed, but it may have been my presence that made him nervous. 'We'll be operating on Mrs Harris tomorrow, she's third on the list,' he said. 'I shall be coming to see her in a moment.'

I hurried over to warn Meg. She got herself ready, straightened her nightdress and gritted her teeth. 'What's he like?' she asked. I said he seemed very nice, very serious. 'Oh I hope he doesn't stare like that other doctor in out-patients. I didn't know where to look. I don't think I'd have cried if he hadn't stared at me so hard. I felt he was trying to tell me something terrible. He was looking at me as if to say, "You know this is it, don't you? You and I know what this means and you haven't got long to live."' I said he hadn't meant that at all. He was a bit frightening but he just wanted to reassure her that nothing was being done behind her back. 'Perhaps,' she answered. 'Anyway you'd tell me what they were saying, wouldn't you?' I said I would, but was secretly determined not to hear anything myself.

The young doctor came over to Meg's bed and discreetly drew the yellow curtains all round it. He began to take her history again from the beginning. He asked all over again almost all the questions the medical student and Mr Thomas had asked in out-patients – a double check.

'When did you first notice the lump?'

'Well, it was two weeks ago. I was getting dressed and I happened to knock my breast with my elbow and it felt funny. I looked at it and felt it and I noticed the lump. It didn't hurt or anything, just felt a funny feeling. But it started to hurt yesterday. Maybe I'm imagining things, but it aches.'

Then the doctor's bleep went. They all carry portable radios with them that bleep when they are wanted. He went to the nearest telephone to find out who was calling him.

'Don't you think it could just be fibrositis?' she asked me. I didn't know what fibrositis was so I just said perhaps.

The young houseman came back.

'I noticed it on the Wednesday,' she said to him. 'I saw my doctor on the Thursday, and he told me to make an appointment here. Well, the soonest appointment they'd give me was for three weeks' time. My husband was really upset and said it wasn't soon enough. So he rang up the appointments people and insisted I get one sooner. They told me a week, so I came up here last Thursday to the out-patients.'

He went through a series of questions. Discharge from the nipple? No. General Health? Good. Heart trouble? No. Get short of breath? No. Ankles swell? No. Palpitations? No. Smoke? Yes. How many? Maybe two a day, never heavily. Any sore throat, cold? No. Ever had TB or chest trouble? No. Appetite? Good. Lost any weight recently? No. Indigestion? Hardly ever. Heartburn? No. Tummy pains? No. Bowels OK? Yes. Waterworks? Yes, except this weekend the nerves affected them. Head-aches? No, only occasional eye-ache. Periods regular? Yes. Painful? Not any longer. No trouble down below?

No. Any joint trouble, back trouble, arthritis? No. Ever had an operation? No, only two babies. Never been in hospital except for the babies? No. Tonsils, appendix, rheumatic fever? No.

Then he asked her about her family's health. She told him about her son's heart complaint. He asked her if there was other heart trouble in the family. 'My sister has a bad heart. She had rheumatic fever as a child, and she's been poorly ever since.' He asked her about her whole family. 'I had three brothers and two sisters. I've lost two brothers.' He asked what they died of. 'One had cancer of the liver, the other I'm not too sure what it was. He had his upper bowel removed but then there were complications and he died. I don't get on with that sister-in-law and she never really explained what the trouble had been. One of my sisters has the heart trouble, but the other's well. Though she had a breast off twenty-five years ago.'

'And she's well now?' asked the doctor taking notes.

'Oh yes. I couldn't tell her I was coming in here though. She'd be too upset, even though she had it done herself. I'm the youngest and they all make a fuss of me. I wouldn't tell the one with heart trouble either as shocks are bad for her — and there might be nothing to worry her about, mightn't there?' she said looking up at him. But he went on writing and refused to be drawn into pronouncing on her chances.

'Do you take any pills or medicines?' he asked.

'Just eye drops for my sore eyes which get inflamed sometimes. And a valium once in a while. I've been taking them this weekend. I got them after my boy was ill. I take one when I start worrying about him too much, when I feel low. No sleeping tablets though.' He asked for her pills and drops and she handed them over. Later he gave them to the nurse who put them in the ward medicine trolley to be dispensed and recorded according to hospital discipline and medical instructions. Anything her GP had prescribed or diagnosed was superseded by the hospital. She belonged, body and soul, to the consultant and his deputies.

'Is your husband well?' asked the doctor. She said he was. He called over a nurse who came in through the curtains drawn around the bed. 'Nurse,' he said starchily – he was young and still embarrassed – 'would you just pop off her things for me. I'd like to examine her.' In hospital everything is 'popped' on or off, 'slipped' in or out. I don't think I met a single doctor who in dealing with patients didn't at some time resort to this sort of nursery talk. I once heard one saying to a patient, an elderly man, 'We're just going to pop you into the operating theatre to have a little peep into your tummy.' Nurses too had people 'popping' all over the place – in and out of lavatories, dressing-gowns, beds, scales, wheelchairs, bandages. I don't think this was through condescension to the patients so much as to cover their own awkwardness and embarrassment. The young doctors used all the same coy phrases, but with less conviction, sounding stilted.

The nurse helped Meg out of her nightdress, carefully covering her up to the stomach with the blankets. 'Now raise that arm – rest the other on my wrist . . . breathe deeply, and rest. Breathe, and rest. Put your arm by your side and press it inwards when I say. Press hard – and rest!' Then he prodded her and she winced. 'Is that a little tender?' (Like a steak?)

She said it was. 'But it's only just started to hurt. It didn't last Thursday when I was examined.'

She looked down at her naked body. 'It looks a bit funny, so brown and so white,' she said, referring to her sun-tan.

The doctor had on his professional face and didn't smile. 'I'm just going to listen to your heart.' He listened. 'Has anyone else in your family had heart trouble?' he asked, looking at her.

She looked suddenly nervous. 'Well, my mother, but she died at eighty-one.'

'Are you sure you never had rheumatic fever?' he asked. She said she was sure, because her sister had it and she'd know if she had too. He made an enigmatic 'Mmm' sound, and she glanced at me anxiously. He listened to her chest and heart again.

'Now I'm just going to test your feet,' he said, and the nurse rolled back the covers. He took out a hammer and scratched the handle along the soles of her feet, which twitched and he said, 'Good.' Then he tapped her knees, which jerked, and she giggled. He asked her to put out her tongue, and he looked in her mouth.

'Can you see which tooth is implanted? It's good, isn't it?' she said.

But he was busy with his examination. He was like a surveyor going over a house for signs of damp or dry rot. There was hardly a corner not tapped or tested by the time he had finished.

'You've never had an anaesthetic before?'

'Only a local one,' she said.

'Well,' he said finally, laying down his tools. 'We'll be operating on you tomorrow. Mr Thomas will be doing the operation, and he'll probably be up to see you later. The anaesthetist will pop in to have a word with you too. You'll be third on the list tomorrow, probably at about eleven o'clock. You know what we're going to do, don't you?' he said to her firmly. She tried to smile and nodded. 'We're going to do what we call a biopsy. We'll take out the lump and send it to the laboratory. When we've got the result of that we know whether we have to go ahead or not.' She said she understood, and he smiled and left her.

I wanted to go after him and ask what he'd found when he examined her. He had kept on about her heart, and had listened to it several times, and kept returning to her family heart history. It made me feel very uncomfortable. As he inspected each part of her he never said, 'That's all right,' or anything reassuring, perhaps because he didn't feel his word was final, as he was only a junior doctor. But he left an unpleasant atmosphere that there *was* something else the matter. I hoped Meg didn't feel the same. But she said almost straight away, 'Do you think he found something wrong with my heart?' I said bravely that I was sure he would have said something if he had, but I wasn't at all sure myself. 'But why didn't he say everything was all right? Why didn't he?' she persisted

Then a girl from Haematology in a white overall came round to take a blood test. I used the time to go and seek out the young houseman, who was still in another part of the ward, out of sight. I had promised myself I wouldn't try to find out anything but I felt I had to know.

I asked him if she was all right. Was there anything the matter with her heart? He looked quite surprised and said there wasn't. I explained that to both of us it seemed as if he had been worrying over it unduly. He said no, everything was fine. I hurried back to tell her.

'He says that was all routine,' I said. 'Nothing at all the matter.'

'Thank goodness. Didn't it give you a turn though?' I said it had.

It occurred to me that all patients in hospital need an advocate, someone to act in their interest, someone not in a nightdress who can ask questions and get answers without fear of offending doctors, getting into their bad books, or being labelled as a neurotic worrier. She would never have dared to ask, in case she'd looked silly, or got a sharp answer, but she would have gone on worrying for a long time. Children in hospital have their mothers with them a good deal of the time, but mothers tend to get treated as patients, as an extension of their children. All patients could do with the protection of a non-patient by their side. Doctors will talk and answer questions much more freely with someone wearing their own clothes, whose life is in their own hands and not in the hands of the hospital.

'I wish they hadn't asked about all my brothers and sisters. Put like that we sound an unhealthy family. I shouldn't think they think there's much hope for me.'

Then a man dressed in white came into the room wheeling a stretcher. A scarcely perceptible hush crept over the ward as everyone looked towards him; he was a kind of angel of death. At first glance I thought he was a doctor, his head wrapped in a white cap, baggy white trousers and a white shirt, operating clothes. But he was only a theatre porter, come to collect the next one on that day's list.

The woman he had come to take was in her thirties and was having a wisdom tooth removed. 'I haven't talked to her myself but the others say she was dreadfully nervous, poor girl,' said Meg. The nurses were helping shift the woman onto the stretcher. She was drowsy, but still awake.

'How does she look, do you think?' Meg asked sitting up in bed watching with a fascinated horror. 'She's not asleep is she? Will I be awake? I couldn't bear to see the operating theatre.'

The woman was wheeled away, and the normal hum of conversation was resumed.

'Perhaps they'll find it's just a muscle out of place,' Meg said. Every so often she kept finding new explanations for her lump, none of which convinced her at all. A physiotherapist came past the end of the bed, helping a very old lady with a walking frame and the bottom part of one leg missing. 'Oh God,' Meg said under her breath. The old woman's empty green pyjama leg was flapping.

A young nurse came bustling along, crisp and perky. 'I'm just going to take your temperature, Mrs Harris,' she said rather too loud, as if she thought the patient stupid or deaf. 'Just pop this under your tongue, dear.' Meg was obedient, and always smiled, eager to please, or at least, anxious not to annoy. Then a set of scales was wheeled in, and she was weighed sitting down, after she'd 'just slipped off' her dressing-gown, and 'just popped' into the chair. 'Now, dear,' said the little nurse, 'is there anything you want to know? Do you understand the visiting hours and everything?' Meg smiled and said she did. The nurse straightened the covers, and hurried away as a team of doctors came breezing into the ward, making people sit up and talk in hushed voices.

There is rarely a spare moment in hospital. Although it is excruciatingly boring, the boredom is ordered and varied, and the patients are kept busy for a good part of the day. Soon another porter came along with a wheelchair to take Mrs Harris to have an X-ray. He was stern and foreign and she was rather abashed when he grabbed her dressing-gown off the bed and shoved it at her. 'This! Put on!' he ordered. And then he wheeled her away.

She was gone for a long time, there being a queue of people waiting for X-rays. I sat by her bed and chatted to some of the other patients. 'I hope she'll be all right,' said the kindly woman next door who had already had a mastectomy. 'She seems so nervous, poor dear. To be honest, it hardly hurts more than an appendix.'

A little later I saw the young houseman again. He must have been thinking about my question about her heart. 'There's clearly some family congenital disorder when so many of them suffer from heart trouble,' he said. He discounted her story that her sister had rheumatic fever, and appeared to disbelieve her son could have had it from tonsillitis.

I went out for a while. The atmosphere in the ward was claustrophobic. I felt oppressed. Or perhaps it was the strain of having to sit all day with Meg, while she agitated and summoned up all her bravery to hide it. I wished there was something, anything, comforting I could say. I was dreading the operation so much myself that I found it hard to look calm and confident, as if I thought it would be all right, when I didn't. On the way back I bought her a bunch of red carnations and blue cornflowers.

When I came back Meg had just arrived from the X-ray department and was more tense than before. 'The anaesthetist came while I was away. I wonder if he'll come back?' She felt it was her fault that she had taken so long. 'Oh dear, I'm sure that X-ray won't come out right and I'll have to have it done again,' she said. 'I was in this big room and they fixed it all up. Then they went out of the room. I heard a voice a long way away saying, "Deep breath!" but I thought it came from another room and they weren't talking to me. The next thing I knew the voice said, "All right, breathe away," and I was already breathing. Do you think it'll come out?'

The tea trolley came round and she had a cup of tea and a small plate of bread and jam. When that was over the ginger medical student came frisking into the ward, with a rather too cheery, 'Hello!' Meg hadn't taken in the difference between doctors and students and referred to him as 'that young doctor who listened so nicely when I came for my first appointment'. He sat down on the bed and asked her how she was. 'Well, sort of nervous. I've never had an operation and I don't like the thought of being put to sleep. It's like dying.'

'No, it's not, not at all,' he said with a laugh. 'It's very restful sleep, with no dreams.'

'When they've taken out the lump,' she said, 'how many days after do they take the whole thing off if they have to?'

He looked surprised by her question and answered at once without realizing how much news he was breaking, 'Oh, but we do it all at once, at the same operation. The surgeon takes out the lump while you're asleep. I'm the runner. I take the lump and I run with it as fast as I can to the laboratory and they examine it. Then they give us the thumbs up or thumbs down. They say whether we have to go ahead or whether there's nothing the matter. If it's yes, and they say go ahead, I come rushing back, and while you're still asleep we take it off, to be sure it hasn't spread anywhere else.'

Meg looked pale, even under her tan. I could hear her gulping, and I could feel her shock. I felt it myself. I had no idea it would all be done at one operation.

'You mean,' she said quietly, 'you really mean that it might happen tomorrow? That when I come round I shan't know if it's there or not?'

'It's always done like that. Really it's to spare you having to go all through it a second time.'

'Well!' Meg said when he'd gone, and that was all.

A woman from across the room came shuffling over, sliding one old bedroom slipper after the other. She was holding a box of Milk Tray in her hand. She always had chocolates with her and ate them all day long. She had fuzzy, pale, mouse-coloured hair, an old candlewick dressing-gown and pop eyes. She was about Meg's age but looked older.

'I've been reading Shirley Temple's story in *Woman's Own*,' she said, starting up the conversation. 'She had one boob off, you know.' This didn't seem to me a very tactful opener, but Meg was kind and felt sorry for her. The woman looked so shabby and down-trodden. 'Shirley Temple says she was always bosomy, like you dear.'

Meg smiled and asked 'What are you in for?'

'Hysterectomy,' said the woman. 'That's why I walk like this. The stitches are killing me.'

'I wish I was having one of those!' Meg said with great passion. 'At least it doesn't show.'

'It's your breast, isn't it?' said the woman. 'You won't believe this but I knew someone had one off. In those days they gave you a falsie filled with sand – a sand bag sort of thing. She was sitting in the pub one night and someone prodded her and the thing bust. Spilled sand all over the floor and her tit went flat as flat. They were looking on the floor and didn't know where all that sand came from!' She handed across her box of chocolates. 'Want one, love?' Meg shook her head and said no, a little frostily, and the woman shuffled away.

Meg took out her handkerchief and blew her nose. 'I feel awful,' she said. 'Oh, I wish it was over. It's the waiting. What am I doing here sitting in bed as if I was dying already, and nothing the matter with me? You know, I think I begin to feel funny already, a bit ill. I feel weak when I get out of bed. That's just from lying down all the time. It's ridiculous!'

It was about six o'clock, and the nurses had started to lay the table in one end of the ward for supper. As the day wore on Meg was getting tired from the tension and anxiety, and the tireder she got, the more depressed she became. She was at low ebb when the Senior Registrar, Mr Thomas came sweeping into the ward, with his small flotilla of juniors, students and nurses. She hadn't yet seen him since that one visit to out-patients.

'Could you just slip your things off as we want to have another look at you,' he said, when the curtains round the bed had been drawn and the whole group were gathered round.

She was surprised to get yet another visit and yet another check. She had no idea of the hierarchy of doctors, and couldn't follow who everyone was, or who was most important. 'I just want to make one last check before the operation,' he said. 'I shan't be seeing you tomorrow, until afterwards. Except of course at the operation, when you won't be able to see me.'

Meg un-buttoned her nightdress. 'It's lucky I bought myself a button nighty,' she said. 'I thought I'd probably have to be examined a lot in it, but not as much as this!' She made a joke of it, but she was especially nervous. She said she found this doctor particularly frightening, perhaps because he was not in the least jolly or facetious, but rather serious. I found him most reassuring and would have preferred his approach to many other doctors, but Meg was unnerved by him. It made her talk a lot.

'Now do you understand what's going to happen tomorrow?' She said she thought she did, and wished it was over. 'We're going to take a look at that lump, take it along to the laboratory and wait until they give us an answer. If the answer is yes, we'll have to take the breast off.'

'Then and there?' she asked.

'Well, it's better, we think, for you to have one operation, not two.' She nodded, looking unconvinced. 'It'll be at about eleven. You'll get a pre-med, a jab to make you drowsy at about ten. Don't expect to be asleep by the time they take you upstairs, because you won't be.' This was good information. Other women in the ward were terrified to find themselves still awake and thought they'd be operated on without anyone realizing they weren't properly under, but they were too sleepy to open their eyes or call out.

Mr Thomas stared at her hard in the eye, and gave her a small smile. She looked back at him, wondering what she should say. He seemed to want her to say something. She looked away, and tears were forming in her eyes again.

'I want a reason, that's all,' she said finally. A tear overflowed and fell down her face. She reached for a Kleenex and wiped it away. 'I want to know *why* it's happening, and why it's happening to me. I keep looking back on the last few years and asking myself what can have caused it. I don't smoke much. I did knock myself not long ago, could it have been that? Did I take too much exercise? I do bicycle a lot. Or perhaps not enough? Couldn't you give me some idea of a reason why it happened to me? . . . No, I suppose you couldn't.'

'I wish we knew. It's just one of those things. We don't know at all at the moment, but perhaps we will some day. You can rest assured that it's nothing you did. You couldn't have prevented it. It's just terrible luck.'

'I haven't told my boys. They know I'm here for something or other. My eldest guessed what it was, but I don't think he realizes I might come home with one breast missing. My youngest doesn't know. How can I tell him?' The tears were falling again.

'Well, perhaps your husband can help. Perhaps he can break it to them gently. But let's not think about it for the moment. You get some good rest for tomorrow.'

'My husband's very good like that. He'll help all he can;' and the thought of her husband brought more tears.

'You'll find you'll hardly notice tomorrow. It'll be come and gone before you know it. It's a funny thing about anaesthetics. You don't have the same sense of time.'

'I can't help thinking about it, doctor. I don't see how I'm going to sleep tonight. I've had a house full of boys and girls all the last few months, sitting around and studying for their O Levels. The place was quite full of kids lounging around, and I was hurrying about getting them coffee and sandwiches I don't know how I could face them, when I come home with one breast. Does that sound crazy to you? I suppose my life style's a bit different to yours,' she said with a nervous laugh.

He coughed and just said, 'Well,' rather quaintly. 'Now,' he said, clearing his throat, 'don't you have any visitors tomorrow. You won't be up to it. Of course your husband can come any time, but no one else.' He started to pull back the curtains, and the interview was over. She had stopped crying, and had a small burst of that strange euphoria that comes after tears.

She didn't even mind when the hysterectomy case shuffled over again, still with her chocolates in her hand. 'They called it a bikini cut, what they've done on my hysterectomy,' she said. She liked rolling the word 'hysterectomy' out, as if it were some smart new possession of hers of which she was proud. 'Can't think why they bothered. A figure like mine I'm not likely to wear any bikini. It's sort of long and curvy, under the tummy. Want to see it?' This last was a joke, not a serious suggestion. Meg smiled. 'I'd still say you were lucky, even if it is painful now,' she said. 'It's better than a breast.' The woman gave her cackling laugh, which showed she'd left out her false teeth, and she moved on.

Meg said she didn't want any supper, but the nurse persuaded her to a bowl of soup. 'You'll be fasting from now on, so you may get hungry later, dear,' she said. Meg asked why, and the nurse explained that anaesthetics make some people sick, so it's better to fast before an operation.

The hysterectomy was cackling in the distance, 'I'm not going to be a martyr to anyone when I get home! Not to my bleeding husband, I can tell you. From now on we'll have to help each other.'

Meg had a wash and got into bed. The night stretched ahead interminably. 'It's only seven,' she said. She was expecting Bob at any moment and he would stay about three-quarters of an hour. 'That's such a short time. Then what shall I do? Will you stay?' she asked. I said I would.

Bob arrived promptly, carrying flowers and some get well cards from friends. One was a beautifully drawn picture of Thor, made by Ian, her younger son. Bob had brought grapes too, but she wasn't allowed to eat anything, so gave them away. I left her for a while and went out to get myself a cup of tea.

The fresh air, the freedom of getting out of that building was intoxicating. By now I felt almost as if I was a patient myself. I had a curious feeling of having escaped, absconded. I decided against tea, and went into the pub over the road for a large drink and a talk with some doctors I knew who were there. I found myself attacking them for callousness and insensitivity – I think unfairly. Patients tend to be over-polite to doctors, through fear of alienating them, but often they feel a curious mixture of overwhelming gratitude, verging on love, and enormous resentment, seeing them as jailers and murderers. As I came out of the pub to go back to Meg I realized I had identified with her case so much that I had been taking it out on these doctors. It was unreasonable, but Meg once said as a joke, 'You get the feeling sometimes that the doctors have invented the illness. Look at me, perfectly healthy. What's a little lump on my breast? Now they're going to put me to sleep, and cut me up, and leave me sore, and hurt and deformed? If you look at it that way, it's them that are doing me the harm!'

On one level, somewhere deep down, I think most patients feel this. 'Why don't you leave me alone? It's all very well for you!' – This attitude towards doctors does come out when things get bad. It isn't a rational desire to be left to die, but a child's healthy resistance to injections or medicine.

Back in the ward Bob had just left. Meg was miserable. She dreaded the night. 'They'll give me a sleeping pill, but I doubt if it'll help. How can I sleep with so much breathing, and snoring and walking around all night?' She took out a photograph of her children and showed it to me. They were two beautiful boys, both with glossy fair hair, long legs and peachy complexions. I said they were lovely. 'They're kind too,' she said. 'I'm lucky. They're very good to me. We have a lot of fun. At least we always have. I don't know about that sort of fooling around fun now, after I've had this, though.'

I began to feel embarrassed at staying in the ward so late. The nurses didn't object but I felt they would rather I left. 'Will you be able to come in the operating theatre with me?' she asked. I said I would. 'Will you be able to bear it? Could you really watch it?' I said I wasn't sure, but hoped so. 'Just you watch they're careful with the knife. Don't let them make fun of me either. No student jokes, mind.' She was trying to be brave, and she was succeeding. She was far braver than I could have been.

Two nurses came around with a medicine trolley, and Meg was given a sleeping pill. I left, and promised to be there in the morning.

I woke at six, at the same time as Meg. I had a night of dreams of all the excuses that might turn up for my not attending the operation. It was a grey morning, misty and dull. I hadn't intended to wake so early. I wished the day was over already.

Meg had slept reasonably well. Nurses came along the ward all night, whispering, muffling giggles, and sometimes shining torches to see that the patients were all right. Meg had cried a little and tried hard to sleep. Her mouth was dry and she longed for a drink but wasn't allowed one.

'I had dreams about going into battle. I thought it was the night before a big battle, and it was silly, but all the women here were soldiers and I knew a lot of us were going to die but I didn't know who. It was a bit like a film I saw once. I don't know if we were men or women,' she said.

She had a bath while everyone had breakfast. She felt shaky. 'I almost wanted to make a run for it. I kept saying to myself, "This is ridiculous. Why am I waiting around here for them to do this terrible thing to me?" I always feel like that about the dentist when I'm waiting. I want to get up and go.'

Meg lay in bed trying to keep calm. It didn't help that her friends in the ward kept coming up to her to wish her good luck, to make jokes and offer odd pieces of advice, but she smiled kindly at them. 'You'll be back in the ward before you know it, just as if nothing at all had happened,' one said. 'Good luck, girl,' said another. 'You've got a lucky face, you'll be OK.' 'You watch out for them young doctors, when they've got you all laid out and helpless!' said a young woman, the coarsest, who always made rude jokes. 'Don't take on, pet,' said the nice lady in the next bed, who had had a mastectomy herself. She patted her hand, and for her comfort Meg was grateful. The kind old deaf lady on the other side beamed at her sympathetically.

'What's it like outside today?' Meg asked. The weather scarcely permeates a hospital, nor does night and day. The hospital routine and moods take the place of weather and time. I said it was grey, and not hot. I didn't say that the streets were full of people selling flags for Cancer Research day. As I had put fifty pence, instead of my usual ten pence, in the tin to ward off danger, I hadn't decided if that was a good or bad omen.

'How do you feel this morning about watching my operation?' Meg asked. I said not too good, but I thought I'd be all right. 'Well, I'm very glad you'll be there. They'll be showing off to you, and they'll make a specially nice job of it, won't they?' she said.

At ten o'clock exactly she was given her pre-med. To her surprise the injection didn't hurt at all. 'I'm really bad about jabs,' she said. 'I tense my muscles and they usually have to more or less screw the needle in.'

She fell very silent very soon, and lay with her eyes shut. 'I'm wide awake,' she kept saying. 'I haven't gone. I'm still here.' She kept licking her lips as if her mouth was very dry. Soon she was far away, and sometimes half muttered something, but her jaw wouldn't open enough to let the words out. She didn't look worried any more. That made me more worried. It was like sitting beside someone who was dying, and I was tempted to shake her awake.

The porter from theatres came to take her away. He was like a mortuary attendant. There was no gleam of interest in his eyes.

Two nurses helped to lift her onto his long trolley, on top of which was a stretcher. Meg murmured. Amongst other things she said, 'I'm really not asleep. I just can't open my eyes or mouth.'

She was too much asleep to notice or mind her operating-gown flapping open; it curled up to her thighs as they moved her. Nor did she feel how clumsily and awkwardly she was handled. Her head flopped back as they put her down.

A young Staff Nurse kept talking to her kindly; soothing, calming words. 'You're all right dear, we're just popping you onto this bed. You'll be fine in a moment. Don't worry about a thing.' Meg gripped her hand tightly. A passing moment of panic? Did she feel she was falling? As the porter pushed her down the corridor to the big lift, she kept a tight grasp of the nurse's hand. Meg's knuckles were white and her nails dug in, but the nurse smiled and said some more soothing things, as she walked along beside her.

Up on the third floor are the operating theatres. They are as old as the hospital itself, and universally considered inadequate, antiquated and not sterile enough. Cracks in the ceilings, walls, and floors give rise to scares about the possibility of infection. The long corridor, lit by sky-lights, from which lead all the theatres, should be a sterile zone, but isn't. People walk in and out of it in their street clothes and shoes. The doors to the theatres swing open and shut into the corridor in the middle of operations.

It is always difficult to assess medical complaints. There are always new machines and new equipment invented which a hospital or a particular department cannot afford. Although the complaints about operating conditions were severe, clearly no one was coming to any harm as a result of them. The infection rate was as low as any other large and important hospital, but even to a layman the theatres did look a bit rugged, primitive and Victorian – far more old-fashioned than other parts of the hospital. This was partly because new operating theatres had been one of the casualties of cut-backs at The London. A whole wing of the hospital had been knocked down ready to house new operating theatres and wards, but the axe had fallen, and the government would not let them proceed with the plan. As new theatres had been expected for so long, not many resources had been spared for modernizing the old ones.

On the same floor, but outside the corridor, runs another long, rickety wooden passage-way, called the 'rabbit warren', for the offices and changing rooms for the theatres. There is a resting room for operating staff, with a constant supply of hot coffee. In there sit groups of exhausted nurses, their white disposable mob caps covering their hair, and doctors in white wellington boots, nasty things that make one feel they've been wading through a floor of blood and gore. This is the only place I found in the hospital where doctors and nurses would actually sit down and drink coffee together. The tension of the operating theatre brought them together, and the rigid segregation was broken down.

The theatre nurses work all day long in the theatres, and not at all in the wards. Most of them do it because the hours are more regular. At night only a handful of them are needed for emergencies. Some of them prefer the work for itself. It is more exciting, there is less drudgery, and less contact with patients and their problems.

One of the nurses in this common room was expecting me. 'Mrs Harris is just resting. She's almost asleep,' she said when she came in. 'They're still on the other case so they won't be doing her for a while.' I asked where Mrs Harris was, and the nurse said she was waiting in the corridor. I remembered Meg saying she didn't like the idea of being wheeled around the place and left waiting in passages with nobody paying any attention to her. I hoped she was too sleepy to know where she was.

The nurse took me to her changing room where she found me a locker to put my clothes in, and gave me a gown, a white mob cap, and big white cloth over-shoes, the kind window-dressers wear. Everything was crisp and hard with starch. The clothes felt dirt-resistant. It worried me that I looked exactly like a nurse or doctor. I clung to my notebook and pencil. I wasn't sure whether I'd be allowed to take such unsterile things into the room, but the nurse smiled and said, 'Of course,' when I asked her. The room was full of unsterile things, like patients' notes and doctors' pens, the trolley the patient was taken in on, and countless other things that caught my eye. I was surprised. The television hospital programmes give the impression that the room contains nothing that hasn't been boiled, except people, and they have been thoroughly scrubbed with carbolic.

When I dressed the nurse took me back to the common room, and we had some coffee. 'Very routine cases on Mr Thomas's list this morning,' she said. I nodded trying to look as if it was routine to me too.

A jolly young West Indian nurse came in. 'This your first?' she asked me. I said it was. 'Will you faint? Most of us did.' I said I hoped not, I didn't faint easily. They laughed disbelievingly.

Mr Thomas came in to get himself a quick cup of coffee before starting on Meg. He gave a nod in my direction, and sank into a chair. Surgeons need good strong legs for all that standing, hours on end. 'That was a nasty hernia,' he said to the nurse beside me. 'Took longer than I'd expected.'

When the nurse and I had finished our coffee, she led me away, down the passage towards the theatres. We went through the swing door into the theatres corridor. There was a lot of coming and going. Everyone seemed to be in a hurry, or exhausted, bustling in and out of the theatres like white ants. Meg was just being wheeled into an ante-room adjoining one of the theatres. There were a lot of people standing round her, but at first it was impossible to tell which were porters or nurses or doctors. She lay there in the little side room where the patient is given the final dose of anaesthetic. Above her head was a big Victorian sky-light, and I saw her eyes open and look up at it for a moment, a little perplexed.

'Hello, Mrs Harris,' said the anaesthetist loudly. 'You don't know me. I came to see you in the ward yesterday but you'd just popped along to X-ray. I'm the one who looks after you for the operation. Can you hear me?' Her head nodded faintly. She looked terrible. Her jaw seemed to have fallen. Her skin was pale and sallow. The bones on her forehead stood out, and she looked older and different, almost unrecognizable. Would she look like that dead?

The anaesthetist pushed me forward and I stood by her head. She opened her eyes for a moment. 'That's you, Polly?' she said.

'How are you?' I asked her.

'Funny,' she said. 'But not asleep, not at all. Tell them.' I told her they all knew she wasn't asleep. 'Have they done it?' she asked. I said not yet, not for a little while. 'Don't go,' she said and seemed to drift away again.

'I doubt if she'll remember any of this. They don't usually,' said the anaesthetist.

He started to give her an injection in the back of her hand. She lay there unchanged. He gave her a short blast of gas, and called her, 'Mrs Harris!' but she seemed before our eyes to sink further down into the bed and the pillow, looking quite flat, as if she was hardly there at all. She looked physically smaller, as if she didn't take up any space, or any thickness.

The same three medical students, the ginger boy and two pretty girls drifted in, all gowned up, and they grinned at me. I was surprised to be recognized by anyone in all that surgical garb. Meg was wheeled through the doors into the adjoining operating theatre, and we all followed her.

The room was light and airy. I was surprised that it seemed much like many other rooms in the hospital. It didn't have a special aura, a sense of drama, or, of meticulous sterility. There was a kind of casualness, people coming and going, talking, sitting about.

The anaesthetist is in charge of a patient during an operation. He controls all the life-support mechanisms, watches the pulse and breathing, tells the surgeon what he can and can't do.

He began to supervise the arranging of Meg on the operating table. The porter helped to move her, together with a nurse. Then the anaesthetist laid her out, arranged for her right arm, on the side that was to be operated on, to be laid out on a plank sideways, and strapped down. A green sheet covered her, through which poked her right breast. The doctors and nurses who were actually assisting at the operation all wore green gowns – the other onlookers (there were two student nurses, as well as the medical students, and one or two other nurses) were dressed as I was, in white. When Meg had been prepared, the anaesthetist sat down on a stool at her head, and there he stayed, watching her for the whole operation, with various machines beside him.

I stood by the door, watching, too terrified to write anything down for the moment. The students stood beside me. They behaved exactly towards me as I expected. The ginger one did most of the talking. 'Mastectomies are the bloodiest of all operations, I always think,' he said gaily. 'Blood spurts out all over the place, very nasty.' One of the girls said, 'I don't know, I've seen one or two that haven't been too messy.'

I asked if they were sure there would have to be a mastectomy. 'Mr Thomas seems pretty sure,' said the other girl.

We were standing by the door, well away from the patient. Other groups of people were standing around talking. Mr Thomas came in, dressed up in green. We were all wearing disposable face masks from a dispenser on the wall of the anaesthetic room. They were hot and scratchy. I was leaning against the wall, holding tight to my notebook. I didn't know when it would start. I hardly dared look. When I did I was glad to find I could barely see. I had hoped that I would be placed behind some viewing panel, well away from the theatre itself. The room seemed small and I wished I was further back.

'Come on,' said the ginger student. 'You can't see here. Come nearer.' Reluctantly I came with them and stood a little behind the surgeon's elbow.

A bright white arc light was beamed down on Meg's breast. It looked curiously splendid, a large firm round hillock all on its own, even defiant. I didn't know when Mr Thomas would start. I couldn't find anywhere else to look. There was still no atmosphere of hush and tension, except inside me and I felt sick and concentrated on appearing nonchalant.

The knife looked like a very small slanted razor blade in a holder. I remembered using one like that to cut cardboard at school, pressing it down and running it along the edge of a ruler to make a perfectly straight incision. He took it up in a matter-of-fact sort of way. I saw him lift it and take it to her breast, and I stepped back without meaning to. I looked at my feet, I looked to one side and to the other, but always out of the corner of my eye I could see what was going on. I couldn't help seeing and I couldn't help not seeing. He held the breast firmly in one hand to stop it moving, and sliced with the other. It wasn't like cutting a cake or carving a joint so much as taking the peel off an orange.

I was surprised and relieved that blood didn't pour or spurt at once. Only a small trickle rolled down her breast like a tear. I could imagine it tickling as it rolled down the side of her body. I looked at it directly and watched the knife approach the nipple. I thought I would faint at once if it even touched the nipple and half gasped. One of the students nudged the others and I clenched my notebook so it suddenly crumpled. But the knife stopped within a millimetre of the nipple.

The skin was peeled back on each side of the cut, again like an orange. The inside was less horrific than the cutting. It was brighter pink and white than I had expected, and not very much blood. The surgeon slid his fingers inside and felt around. The blood made nasty vein-like tracings on his cream rubber gloves. He began explaining to his young houseman, and the student nurses in front of him what he was doing. I couldn't hear what he said although I was close. The words were a noise that didn't register sense in my brain. It went on a long time.

With a small pair of scissors he started to cut away at a piece of tissue. The sound of the snipping was as bad as the sight of the knife. He felt around and snipped, slowly and steadily, pulling at a piece of flesh. It didn't look any different from any other bits inside the breast – not a noticeably different round lump, as I had imagined. It felt different to his touch, not his eye. I was only looking in glances and didn't see exactly. He was talking, still in an ordinary everyday voice – no hush or special reverence. 'You notice it's unexpectedly pale,' he said as he eased out a bit more. It was a great pink mass he was lifting and snipping out of the breast, almost as big as the palm of his hand.

I don't remember the words, but it dawned on me slowly

what he was saying. I thought I hadn't understood. I began to listen. I still didn't know if I had understood – but I had.

As he finally lifted the flabby pink lump from out of her breast, with a last snip, he was sure. 'We won't bother to send it to the laboratory.' he was saying. 'I'm absolutely sure, just from looking at it. We'll send it along later just as a final check, but I'm quite sure.'

I turned quickly to the students, to be certain that I had understood what he was saying. 'What's he mean?' I whispered.

'It's all right!' said one of the girls, breaking into an enormous smile. Then everyone in the room, the surgeon too, was smiling and looking pleased. It wasn't cancer, and she was going to be fine!

The pleasure on their faces was a surprise and a delight. They were really, genuinely very pleased and very happy. Most of the people in that room had never seen or heard of Meg Harris until she was wheeled into the theatre, looking like a not-quite-human thing that morning, and yet they had cared – not just that a good job should be done, but they cared that her breast should be saved, and possibly her life. I had misjudged them. The calm and uninvolved way in which the operation was carried out had led me to believe that they all regarded her as just number three on the list, just another probable mastectomy case. It wasn't their own skill that had made them so pleased, but the fact that they weren't going to have to use it after all. I would have expected a moment of euphoria at the end of a difficult heart by-pass operation, a celebration of their own tremendous surgical prowess, but here was everyone being pleased because Meg didn't have cancer. Even the students were moved and pleased, even the student nurses, even the hardened operating theatre Sister. Did they have time to be pleased or sad at the end of every operation every day? I think they probably did.

It only lasted a moment, a brief sigh of relief and pleasure. Then, still holding the lump in his hand, Mr Thomas leaned over Meg to show it to everyone and to explain how he knew it was harmless. He sliced it open, and said it was white and pulpy, had liquid inside, was not a sinister dark grey. It was a complete surprise, quite unexpected. Externally there had been all the characteristics of malignancy. He dropped it into a silver dish and it was left to one side to be sent to the laboratory later.

Mr Thomas set about sewing up the wound, after swabbing and cleaning it. The needle piercing the flesh was an ugly sight, but nothing seemed very bad now. Her large bright nipple still stood there safely on top. There seemed to be a slight dent where the lump had been, but not a large one. The line of stitches, when completed, looked unreal, as if it was a plastic scar that could have been peeled off like a piece of sticking plaster. The dark line and darker knots made a cruel contrast with the white of her breast, but nothing seemed too bad now.

I wondered what was going on in her mind. She wouldn't remember, but was she still worrying inside there somewhere? I wanted her to wake up at once, to sit up and see that her breast was still there.

When it was all over and she was cleaned up, there was still a small smear of blood down her side, where the first drops had fallen. She was wheeled away to the recovery room. It wouldn't be long before she reached some kind of consciousness.

I left the room. My legs felt odd. I must have been standing with them quite stiff and they felt strange to walk with. I went back to the changing room, opened my locker with the key on the string round my neck, threw off the operating clothes into the big laundry basket and dressed quickly. The nurse had advised me not to see her until she was back in the ward, so I left the hospital. The grey misty morning had turned hot again. I looked at my watch for the first time, and it was twelve o'clock. It had all taken only an hour, but it felt like all day. I bought another flag for Cancer Research.

Sitting in the Underground train on the way back to my office I looked numbly at the other passengers and thought how thin their skin was, how much was going on underneath it, how little most of us know about our own bodies. All that flesh and rawness seemed barely covered up. I didn't like the feel of my own body or the look of anyone else's. Do surgeons find people disgusting? What can Mr Thomas feel when he touches a breast, only lumps and layers, tissues and blood? Does it change your view of the world and of people to be a surgeon? I never managed to ask that question of any of them in a satisfactory way; at least I never got a good answer.

Meg opened one eye in the recovery room, she told me afterwards, and a nurse with curly hair was leaning over her shouting, 'Mrs Harris! You've still got it, Mrs Harris!' at the top of her voice, or so it seemed. She had no idea what the woman was talking about and wished she'd leave her in peace to sleep. Then it seemed like a long time afterwards, it dawned on her. She remembered all about everything, and she understood that she'd still got her breast. Her arms felt too heavy to lift, but she wanted to touch it to make sure. When she did all she could feel was a bandage, and wondered if it was true, or if they might have just told her that to make her get better sooner. She was suddenly back in the ward, and couldn't remember how she got there.

Bob came to see her. She talked on the telephone to her elder son, who had just taken his first two O Levels. He told her he thought he'd done very well in both. Her younger boy sounded cheerful, and the doctor said she'd be able to go home quite soon. Her stitches didn't hurt but she didn't dare move her arm for fear of pulling them.

She was still very sleepy when I saw her. The effects of the anaesthetic lasted a long time. When I talked to her she was drowsy, and her sentences were sometimes disconnected, and sometimes tailed away altogether. She smiled and beamed and slept. She still seemed far away. Bob was euphoric, couldn't stop talking, but he was alarmed by her oddness and her seeming to be somewhere else, on another plain. She looked ill, still looked close to death. She still melted into the pillow her head rested on. Her tanned face was still sallow and sunken, and her bones protruded. I didn't stay long, and she slept most of the day.

But the next day the change was astonishing. I came in at ten o'clock in the morning, twenty-four hours after the operation and she was sitting bolt upright in bed, chatting to another patient, laughing, and quite transformed. The colour was back in her cheeks. She looked round and healthy, not drawn, and above all she looked happy. She looked like young mothers are supposed to look after having a first baby. She looked younger than her forty-six years. Before she had seemed strange and extraordinary, ethereal and mysterious, now she was ordinary, and like other people again.

'Today I can hardly remember anything at all,' she said with a laugh. 'I can hardly remember yesterday. It was gone before I knew it. I do remember the nurse telling me I still had it. I hope never in all my life to forget that moment. I felt such gratitude, just for being alive.'

She asked what the operation was like, though she didn't ask and I think didn't want to know much about the details. So I told her how delighted they'd all been when they found it wasn't cancer, and how touching it was. 'Isn't that nice?' she said, quite moved as well. 'They really bothered to be pleased?' I told her that it wasn't just Mr Thomas and the young houseman who had met her, but that all the theatre staff who hadn't were so relieved too. 'They are such good people, aren't they?' she said. 'Such very good people.' I agreed.

I asked her what else she remembered. 'I kept saying, "I'm sorry" to the anaesthetist at first, because I couldn't keep my eyes open when he was talking to me,' she said. 'My husband says I always apologize too much, that I'd say sorry if someone trod on my toe. I was left in a corridor, wasn't I?' I admitted that she was. 'I was just parked by a wall for a time?' I said yes. 'Then they took me into the operating theatre, and I was still awake. I opened my eyes and there was a big window in the ceiling, and the sun was shining on it. Am I imagining that?' I said that she had been put under a big sky-light, but that was in the little anaesthetic room, next to the theatre itself. 'Were you there? Did I see you? Oh yes! I remember you were there, with a face mask on, and a white hat. You smiled and I held your hand. I can't remember seeing anyone else. I can't remember the recovery room either. The first thing I can think of now is turning my head very slowly to the right and seeing that window over there, in the ward, with the green trees outside, swishing about in the wind. I knew I was back in the ward by that window, and I knew I was alive. I thought they hadn't done anything to me yet. Then the Sister came up to me and said, "You know you've still got it, don't you, dear?" I did know by then, but I forget who first told me. A nurse shouted it at me, but I can't think when or where. Just the words, "You've still got it", will always stick in my mind.'

Today Meg wanted to talk and talk. Everything she had felt and thought came tumbling out. Her worst fears, now they were over, were easy to talk and laugh about. She darted from one thing to another and scarcely drew breath.

'It was so terrible, that night before the operation,' she said. 'I tossed and turned, and I imagined the lump hurt. I don't know if it really did, but the pain was dreadful all night. It got so I kept saying to myself, "I'll be glad when they take the flipping thing off and have done with it." Everyone was asking for valium that night. I had one, but I could have done with a couple. I woke up at four in the morning and didn't go to sleep again. I was glad they got us up so early then, except the time dragged until ten. I had a bath. I lay there looking at my boob and feeling sorry for my husband, and I cried. I felt the cancer was like a lobster growing in me, like Cancer the sign of the Zodiac.'

The deaf old lady in the next bed was being encouraged to eat. 'Some lovely trifle with chocolate and chopped nuts, dear?' one of the nurses shouted at her.

'Ooh yes, love,' said the woman, taking off her specs and putting down her magazine. 'Aren't the meals wonderful in here?' she said to Meg and I. Meg smiled and agreed.

'Glad she thinks so,' she said quietly to me. 'These poor old people, I don't suppose they bother cooking for themselves at home, so it probably does seem a treat to them.'

Meg hadn't been able to eat her lunch. 'It was kidney soup,

and it smelled of you-know-what, pardon the expression,' she said, making a face. 'Then we had what they had the nerve to call "Sauté of Chicken", a pale grey thin mince.' She took a drink of lemon squash from beside the bed.

'My sister used to say she had breast cancer all those years ago because they forced her to breast-feed, even when it hurt and she had to use a nipple shield. They did ask me if I breast-fed. I fed both my boys. Do you think it was because of that I got a lump?' I had asked the doctor why they'd asked Meg if she'd breast-fed. He said that no one yet knew whether there was any connection. Some had said that breast-feeding stopped cancer, others that it caused it. As yet, he said, there was no proper evidence one way or the other, so they were collecting it.

'You'll think it silly of me now, but I thought when I came in here on Monday that I might never come out alive. So on Friday I went down to the Halifax Building Society and changed the money from my name to my husband's. My brother left me £600 when he died. I remember when my father died my mother had a terrible time getting the money out, as it was in his name, so I just thought I'd put that right. The same morning Bob and I went shopping. I wanted a couple of new nighties to come in here with. We were walking through Woolworths and I saw some big foam-rubber-filled bras. I said to him, "I'd better have one of those!" I was brave enough to make jokes.' She sipped at her glass.

'Bob didn't like it, and I saw he looked upset. You know, I bet you anything when I go home that bath rail will be fixed! He's been meaning to do it for two years, and I bet you he's done it now! Oh yes, I gave Bob the mould for my implanted tooth. I said to him, "Here it is if they break my tooth in the operation. You go and get me another one made." I thought of everything, I can tell you.'

A physiotherapist came by, helping the same one-legged old lady with a walking frame. 'Look up, dear!' she was saying. 'You know, that floor must be very interesting, the way you're staring at it!' We watched quietly for a moment.

'We're not at all prudish, our family,' Meg said. 'We walk about without clothes, but I was thinking to myself all that would have to change. I'd have to keep well covered up. I was in a terrible state. I cried over the least thing all weekend. I even said prayers, and I don't know how to pray!'

The gentle woman who had comforted Meg before the operation, and who had had a mastectomy herself, came and sat by us. She showed not the slightest jealously at Meg's good luck. I'm so happy for you, dear,' she said, and beamed at her. They were giving an injection to a younger woman across the room who was due to be operated on that morning.

'Poor thing!' said Meg with real feeling. 'She was terrified, I think even more afraid than I was. She's got a lump too, but the doctors told her there was a good chance it wasn't cancer. They never told me that, so she'll probably be all right.' I said different doctors tended to tell their patients different things. 'We have no modesty in here,' Meg said. 'She showed me her lump to see what I thought. It was much smaller and harder than mine. She was glad it was smaller, as she thought that was a good sign, but it worried her that it was harder than mine. The doctor said at her age, mid thirties, it wasn't so likely to be cancer as at mine.'

The hysterectomy, with another box of chocolates, shuffled across to join us. 'Another one for the chop!' she said, nodding towards the woman to be operated on. She offered us all chocolates which none of us accepted.

An old lady was brought back from the operating theatre coughing all the way down the passage. We could hear her in the distance. As soon as she had been lifted back to her own bed she began to be sick, over and over again.

'What a shame!' said Meg. 'They shouldn't bring her back in that state.'

'They could at least put curtains round her, couldn't they?' said the mastectomy.

'I think it's disgusting,' said the hysterectomy, still chewing chocolates.

It was indeed a very distressing sight, the poor frail old

woman green and harrowed, hardly conscious, retching and coughing in turns. You could hear the pain.

'She snores badly,' said the hysterectomy. 'Kept me awake last night.'

A doctor hove into the room and went from bed to bed examining the charts. He looked at the one at the end of Meg's bed, said nothing and moved on. None of us had seen him before, and he never said who he was, but left the ward again. A great many mysterious things happen in hospital that no one bothers to explain. Patients in a state of anxiety about their health, which Meg was no longer, look for all kinds of meanings in these odd happenings.

A nurse brought in a very young girl and showed her to her bed. She looked about thirteen or fourteen, dark, shy and pretty. The curtains were pulled round her while she undressed.

'She's too young to be in here, with the likes of us,' said the hysterectomy. 'We won't do her any good!' and she gave her usual crackly laugh.

'Poor lamb!' said the mastectomy. 'She should be with the kiddies.'

When the girl's curtains were drawn back and she was in bed, her father came to sit by her. He was a rabbi in a big black hat and beard. Both of them looked appalled at the sight of this strange collection of middle-aged and elderly ladies staring back at them. They smiled nervously and several women smiled back kindly. Some of them were wearing curlers, one in the next bed to the girl was eating an orange and the smell wafted down the ward. The girl was holding her father's hand and looked close to tears.

I had to go, but when I came back later Meg said the young houseman had seen her, and Mr Thomas too, and that she would be released the next day. She had stopped thinking about hospital and the other patients. Now she was only thinking about going home.

'I don't think I can stand another night in here. I can't breathe. All I can think of is getting out, having a good meal and seeing the boys,' she said.

She made elaborate plans, folded and refolded her things ready for packing. The others in the ward looked at her with envy. Now she had been given a time, ten o'clock tomorrow, she was, in their eyes, already a part of the outside world. She didn't quite belong any more to their little enclave.

'Oh, I'd give anything to be you,' said one. 'Just to walk in the street!' said another. 'I'd love to go shopping, choose what I want,' said a third.

Meg began to be like a visitor, not a patient. 'I'm sure you'll be fine, out and about in a few days! You'll be right as rain in no time! Oh they won't keep you long, now you're doing so well!' she said cheerily to them all, the ill and reasonably well alike.

'They're not taking my stitches out until next week. I've got to come back to have them out in out-patients, so I'll drop by and see you all,' she promised.

The night ahead stretched out as long as the night before her operation. 'There's one silly thing I forgot to tell you,' she said, as I was going. 'Did you notice I had quite a bit of make-up on for my operation? I spent a long time doing it. I know it's silly, but I thought if I looked really nice they'd care more, and do a specially good job on me!'

The nurses too treated Meg differently once she had been given a definite time to go home. She was not really ill any more, and hardly belonged to them. In a way she began to feel a little excluded from the camaraderie of the ward – though excitement at going home filled most of her thoughts.

'I shall miss some of the friends I've made here,' she said next morning, an hour before Bob was due to come and collect her.

'I'm going to do everything for her, everything! Nothing's too much for her,' Bob said, as he waited outside the ward. He was beaming, and for the first time looked confident. At all his other visits he had been sheepish, awkward, shy of the nurses and alarmed by the other patients. Now he was going to take Meg home, it was all over, and he was so pleased that he couldn't stop smiling. He grinned at the nurses, the doctors, the cleaners, the porters, as they came past him in the corridor outside the ward.

Leaving hospital is a difficult thing to do gracefully, leaving behind the friends that have become compulsory intimates in a short time, knowing you will probably never see any of them again, that you are free and they are still trapped. It's a moment that chills the hearts of the other patients – an empty bed, and soon a new face.

Meg pulled the curtains round the bed while she dressed and put her last few things into her suitcase. She'd been fiddling around with her packing since seven o'clock that morning. She poked her head out of the curtains and handed her two vases of flowers to the deaf lady. Her chocolates and grapes she gave to her other neighbour. She finally shut her case and pulled back the curtains. There she was, transformed from the woman they all knew, in her familiar dressing-gown, to a strange person from the outside, in clothes they didn't know, her hair smart, her face made up. It often surprises people to see patients in their street clothes, as they suddenly seem like a different sort of person. Meg was quietly, elegantly dressed, with a neat coat over her arm. Sometimes patients who have seemed quiet and mousy emerge in bright and garish clothes loud make-up and high hair styles, upsetting at the last moment, everyone's impression of them. Husbands and relatives too often come as a surprise. Some of the women in the ward talked all the time about their husbands, but when they actually turned up they were quite different from what everyone had imagined.

Meg managed her good-byes and her exit with great tact. She looked a little embarrassed, a little regal and very friendly, as she went round each person wishing them luck. Most of her warmth was reserved for her two neighbours.

The deaf lady smiled and held her hand firmly. 'I'm so glad for you, dear, that it all turned out so well. Don't you worry about me. I like it here. Such a nice place.'

The woman with the mastectomy held her hand too and smiled affectionately. Meg was a little lost for words. What comfort could she offer? 'You've been so good to me. If it had been me I couldn't have been brave like you,' she said.

'Oh nonsense,' said her friend. 'It really isn't so bad when it actually happens. You had the worst of it, the waiting, and the going into the operation.'

Meg said a last good-bye to the whole room, and in a moment was gone.

There was a small silence.

'Lucky bugger,' said a young woman at the other end of the ward.

'You'll be home soon too,' someone answered.

Two auxiliary nurses came to change Meg's bed, to wash down her locker with disinfectant, to remove every trace of her. I sat for a little while chatting to one or two of the women. Soon there was no sign that Meg had ever been there.

'Wonder if there's someone else coming in today?' someone asked.

'Bound to be. With waiting lists the way they are, they never leave them empty long,' someone else said.

'Hardly time to let a bed go cold!' said another woman.

Meg found Bob outside the ward and she gave him the case to carry. She had said many grateful good-byes to the nurses. It happened that the houseman was around to thank, but she wished she could have seen Mr Thomas once more. 'I'll send the nurses a present, maybe a big tin of biscuits. I've heard that's what they like for their coffee breaks,' she said.

'We'll send them ten tins if you like,' said Bob, still grinning. He was edging her towards the lift, anxious to be away. We said our good-byes and I watched them go.

The lift arrived, and a very old lady with a bad limp came out. She walked with the aid of a stick in one hand, and the support of a balding middle-aged man on the other, perhaps her son. Meg and Bob got into the lift, we waved, and the doors shut on their beaming faces.

Slowly, painfully, the old woman edged down the corridor towards the ward. Just behind them was the same lady from the admissions office in her salmon pink overall. We recognized one another and smiled. 'She gone then?' she asked. I was surprised she remembered, I said she had.

'Mr Hastings, would you just sit your mother down here for a minute while I go in and see that they're all ready for her?' she said to the man in her sugary voice. He carefully sat his mother down on the same bench that Bob and Meg and I had waited on. It seemed so long ago now, the waiting, the agonizing. By the time she left I think Meg had managed to forget it too. It had all been just a minor operation, of no significance, just five days in hospital, and a small scar to show for it.

The following Thursday Meg didn't go back to see her friends in the ward. She was kept waiting so long in out-patients that she had to hurry home. She was glad in a way. She wasn't sure anyone would have remembered her, and now she was out, she wasn't sure that she'd have anything at all to say to them.

4

Nurse

Anne French was a Staff Nurse on Talbot Ward – men's surgical. She was in her twenties and had worked on the ward for six months. It was her second staff job since she passed her finals and qualified as a State Registered Nurse. She trained at The London. She was now considering taking a six-month specialized course in the Intensive Therapy Unit. She was a serious intense girl, timid but with great firmness under her apparent shyness. She thought carefully before she spoke.

One of the surprising things about her was that she had few academic qualifications. To be accepted for training at a famous teaching hospital like The London, it is usual for nursing applicants to have about five O Levels and two As. She had only three Os and a CSE in typing, but it does credit to the nursing selectors that they looked beyond her paper qualifications and saw the makings of an excellent, dedicated and intelligent nurse.

There are two stereotyped views of nurses. One says they are angels of mercy, sweetness and self-sacrifice; the other that they are tough, insensitive and either frivolous or ferocious. Most people who have been in hospital come out with one version or the other. What neither picture allows is that they might also be clever. I felt a good many of the nurses I met were equal in intelligence, and occasionally in status to some of the doctors.

The rigidity of the barrier between doctors and nurses is the first principle grasped by every patient within half an hour of entering the hospital doors. The affronts to the nurses by some of the older and more insufferable consultants are numerous, and the casual conceit of some of the more insecure younger doctors is often in evidence. But what it takes longer to observe is the extent to which these barriers are breaking down, and the respect with which nurses are regarded by the more enlightened doctors, who ask their opinions and listen carefully to what they say, since the good nurses often know far more about the state of their patients than the doctors do. Often young doctors have to depend greatly on the knowledge and experience of specialized nurses, and openly ask them questions about treatment. Newly arrived doctors, ignorant of the intricacies of some specializations are firmly put in their place unless they recognize the real value of the Staff Nurses and Sisters.

It may not be fair to generalize about nurses from meeting those at a teaching hospital, which can afford to select none but the best. (One difference that strikes one immediately, and when inquired about receives curiously evasive replies, is that, given the very high number of coloured and immigrant nurses who keep the health service going, The London's nurses, as at the other teaching hospitals, are almost entirely white.)

Anne French is a small slight girl, with fairish hair, looped back in a bun. She wears the purple uniform of Staff Nurses, pretty and becoming. The nurses' uniforms at The London are among the most old-fashioned, and beautiful of any in the country. They have huge puffed starched sleeves, come well below the knee, and are made of thick crisp cotton. The student nurses wear mauve checks, the Staff Nurses purple stripes, and the Sisters a pretty mid-blue. The hats are tiny, white and tucked, pinned precariously on the top of the head. The Sisters' hats are laced and frilled. On high days and holidays they add long white tails to them, reaching to their waists, like Victorian parlour maids. All the nurses have crisp white aprons, which they wear only in the ward, a sign of being on duty. They have to take them off for meal breaks. The uniforms are covered in buttons, but are in fact held together almost entirely by clips or pins. The buttons have to be taken off to go to the laundry, so they are safety-pinned on instead of sewn. All the uniforms are short-sleeved, though the Sisters have some rather odd-looking sleeves which they have to pull on, like opera gloves, whenever they leave the ward. This was originally because the Sisters, as a sign that they didn't do much dirty work, had long sleeves, which they would roll up to work in, and unroll as they left work. Detachable sleeves are apparently more practical. The uniform, for all its fiddliness to wear, is enormously popular. I never heard anyone express anything but delight with it. It was even suggested that many girls, not knowing how to choose between hospitals to train at, came to The London on account of it. Even the manager of the hospital laundry, who had the terrible job of organizing the ironing and pleating and goffering and starching, was immensely proud of the uniform, and viewed with contempt the little nylon-mix uniforms that have been substituted in the name of practicality and hygiene in many hospitals. He says these nylon uniforms are much less hygienic as they cannot be boiled. All his uniforms are boiled twice a week. There is a special machine called Big Bertha which presses the Sisters' uniforms by inflating them.

Anne French had reached the level of seniority where she could come off the rota system worked by more junior nurses. This meant that she no longer had to do night duty. She worked one of two shifts, eight in the morning to four o'clock in the afternoon, or one-thirty in the afternoon to ten o'clock at night. She worked a cycle of ten days' work, followed by four days off, then eleven days' work followed by three days off. She was supposed to work a forty-hour week, but in fact, for all nurses the hours are much longer. Reclaiming the extra hours worked is almost impossible, as the wards are so busy most of the time. She is curiously vague about how much she earns. The computation of hours and special duty payments is so complex that when she gets her pay slip she has only the roughest idea of whether it is right. Occasionally mistakes are made, she says. 'The money really doesn't worry me, as long as it's more or less accurate. I don't do the job for the money.' A large number of the nurses I met had this sort of attitude towards pay. Perhaps this is because nurses are better paid now than they used to be, or perhaps they were never as militant as they were protrayed by some unions. However, she thinks she probably earns about £120 a month, after tax and deductions (about £2000 a year gross).

Talbot Ward is modern with a T-shaped layout. There is a corridor where the nurses' desk is placed, and three partitioned sections each containing four beds. At the end of the corridor, across the top, is a long light room with twelve beds in it. There is an atmosphere of quiet and calm. Nobody runs, or even bustles. How this atmosphere in the ward was maintained was something of a mystery to me. The nurses are in fact working at a frenetic speed, hurrying from one job to another, constantly interrupted, and having to remember a long list of things to be done at any one time. They are having to sort out their priorities and do the most important things first, making sure that some things don't get left out altogether. For the senior nurses there is a considerable amount of report-writing, requisitioning, and paperwork of all different kinds. Each time they go on and off duty they have to re-familiarize themselves with the patients, who are constantly coming and going, being admitted or discharged, getting better or worse.

I set out to follow Anne French around wherever she went, to listen to every conversation she had with doctors, patients and colleagues. For her, I am sure, I was something of a cross to bear. Being shadowed for every minute of the day can't have been easy, but she was patient. It wasn't easy either on my feet. She said that at first young nurses suffer dreadfully from never sitting down, and that still her feet and legs often ached unmercifully. This I could understand, after a day or two following her. I have no idea how many miles she walked, but it must have been plenty.

Talbot Ward, it turned out, specialized mainly in bowel operations, which I hadn't realized before I went to spend some time there. There were also some ENT cases (ear, nose and throat), a few dental cases, a fractured jaw, and one or two other minor surgical cases. The men's ages ranged from sixteen to seventy the week I was there. The average age of patients in surgical wards is younger than that of patients in medical wards. The bowel surgery patients were mostly suffering from some form of intestinal cancer. I thought this must be one of the worst nursing jobs in the hospital, both in being most depressing, and one of the messiest jobs. But Anne said that in her view it wasn't. 'Each speciality has its nasty side,' she said. She had disliked midwifery, and had found caring for leukaemic patients more upsetting. She said that the medical wards, with many more elderly patients, involved more bed pans and cleaning up as more patients were incontinent and incapable of feeding themselves. It seems that all nurses have different sensibilities and squeamishnesses, which is just as well, since all the jobs have to be done. I could never imagine myself as a nurse. I found it hard to understand them, to put myself in their shoes or to see what made them do it. As a result I had to fight off the temptation to dismiss them as being saints, or in some important way, less sensitive than I. But the truth, I think, is that they are just different. And of course, squeamishness is something we can all overcome in a very short time indeed, given an environment like a hospital where it just doesn't exist. By the time I had finished my tour of the hospital there were a lot of things I could contemplate and discuss calmly that made my friends turn white and green.

This chapter shows something of the chaos of hospital life – the thousands of small chores, conflicting duties and things to be remembered. A day in the life of a ward is hard to describe, as seen from a nurse's viewpoint, as it is a collection of running stories and events overlapping and interrupting each other. Small things and important things crowd together in too-quick succession to show hardly more than the random little scenes that tumble out one after another all day long. In all the apparent chaos the good nurse is the calm centre making some kind of order out of it all, remembering everything while distracted by so many conflicting things that need to be done at any one time. One of the things that struck me most forcibly was how little time there was for a nurse to establish any but the most fleeting relationships with her patients. She cannot sit soothing brows and listening to woes for more than a fraction of the time. She does not know her patients well. And yet the good nurses manage to establish friendly and trusting relationships with their most needy patients in just a few minutes' conversation a day. It's a talent Anne French had. She said she didn't feel she really knew any of them, yet I felt that some of the illest ones regarded her as a friend.

On Monday Anne French came on duty at one-thirty in the afternoon. That week the ward Sister was away on holiday and a new relief Sister was in charge, who had only been at the hospital two months, and was still a little uncertain about the running of some things. This meant that Anne, as her deputy, had a little more work and responsibility than she would normally have had.

The previous shift, with no Sister, but another Staff Nurse in charge, were still frantically busy, too busy to stop work and hand over to the on-coming shift. The official handover comes when the senior nurse on one shift addresses the senior nurse and her juniors on the next and reads over a full report on the state and requirements of every patient in the ward. But there was no time for a report at once, so Anne set to work clearing up and sorting out the mess in the dressings room, where all the sterile supplies are kept in boxes.

Then she went to help the departing Staff Nurse with the last part of a round dispensing drugs. There have to be two people to check each dose as it is administered to double-check for any error. A little first-year student nurse was passing. 'Would you give Mr Henderson an enema, Nurse,' asked the Staff Nurse. The girl looked anxious. 'Haven't you done one before? Do it with Maria and she'll show you,' she said, and the girl hurried away. The drug round was finished and the drugs trolley was wheeled away and padlocked to a pillar.

It was then time for the report. All the nurses on the new shift drew up chairs and stools to the nurses' desk, and the departing Staff Nurse balanced a Kardex file on her knees. She talked quietly, and Anne and the others leaned towards her to hear what she said. She was thorough and went over the medical histories of even those patients who had been in the ward a number of weeks, for the benefit of the new nurses.

'Mr Singh needs a pump on his drain. . . . Mr Simpson with the rectal prolapse had a good day. . . . Mr Weston with an acoustic neuroma is having a lumbar puncture later today. . . . Mr Evans, carcinoma of the caecum had a rectal lavrage this morning. . . . Mr Morley with gangrene of the great toe and iscaemic disease has had a comfortable day. . . . Mr Hatch, meningitis needs a bit of help walking as he came to grief this morning. . . . Mr Harris has a pain in his left side from the nylon suture. . . . Mr Carter, age seventy, sigmoid carcinoma seems very confused today though, he was all right yesterday.'

Anne interrupted. 'Oh, that's a shame. He was doing so well. I talked to him a lot yesterday and he wasn't at all confused then.'

'Well, it seems to come and go. Sometimes he seems to make sense but I don't think he really knows where he is or what's going on at the moment,' the other Staff Nurse said, and Anne nodded.

'Mr Perrin complains that he has been hallucinating on and off. The medical staff saw him about it this morning but I don't think they realized how bad it was. They've decided to take him off all the anti-depressant drugs for the moment to see if that makes it better, but he's now suffering more pain. . . . We are about to admit a Mr Rabkin, aged thirty-nine with a perianal abscess. . . . Last night we admitted a Mr Shona with a fractured mandible. He had it wired in theatres today and he is now on half-hourly observations. His pupils are unequal, but apparently that could be long-standing, from a car crash he had some years ago. We're trying to check with the hospital that he was in before he was transferred here to see if they noticed it. . . . Mr Garside, aged fifty-three, has been transferred here from

George Ward with carcinoma of the rectum. He has had a barium enema and ECG. He is on the fluid diet from now on. He will start rectal lavrages from tomorrow. He says he fell over last night and banged his head. A nurse was there and says he didn't seem to have hurt himself. He hasn't mentioned it since. We have just admitted a Mr Grover, a twenty-eight-year-old with haemorrhoids, for theatres tomorrow. . . . Mr Champion may be going home at the weekend. He is managing his colostomy well, but needs encouragement. We must assure him how well he's doing, so he knows he'll manage all right when he gets home.' That was the end of the report, and the tired Staff Nurse went off.

Quietly, while they were still sitting round the desk, as the Staff Nurse on duty, Anne French gave out particular tasks to each of the students. It was the Staff Nurse who was responsible on this occasion for deploying the available labour in the ward.

A sweet-looking, large and dumpy nurse was given the job of admitting the new patient who was waiting outside the ward. Another girl was given the responsibility of the half-hourly observations on the unconscious man with the broken jaw, and the other two were sent off on other jobs. Anne herself chose the important job of talking to and assessing the two patients who seemed, since her last shift, to have had most emotional upset.

First she went over to Mr Perrin, the man who had complained of hallucinating. He was a middle-aged man with grey hair, and a pale grey complexion. He was lying listlessly on his bed wrapped in a blue quilted dressing-gown, attempting to concentrate on the *Daily Telegraph*. There was a sad, almost despairing look about him. She sat down quietly by his bed, and he put down his paper. She talked in a low voice to him for some time. He described the hallucinations, and she nodded, and discussed with him which pills it might be that caused it. But he seemed so gloomy, perhaps partly because he had slept little the night before. She talked to him for about five minutes, and he smiled briefly as she came away.

'He's a frightened man, I'm afraid,' she said to me in explanation. 'He's a dying man. Does he know it? Well, he could if he wanted to, if you see what I mean. He has all the information. I'm sure he suspects but perhaps isn't able to face up to asking direct questions. He won't live very long. His painkilling drugs are not being effective and he feels a lot of pain. Something more should be done for him.' A young doctor came up to her and she said she thought Mr Perrin ought to have more painkiller. He looked at the patient's notes and shook his head. 'He's had all those drugs before, and they didn't make him hallucinate then. Which ones does he think cause it?'

'The pink or the brown, he says.'

The doctor nodded and told her to give him a larger dose for the pain. 'By the way,' he said, as she turned away, 'do you happen to know the maximum dosage for this?' She looked at the drug he was pointing at. She thought about it and said she wasn't absolutely certain, so he went to check.

Then two other doctors came into the ward. They were neuro-surgeons who had come to see Mr Hatch, a twenty-three-year-old who had been operated on to try to correct severe trembling of the body, due to a serious case of tubercular meningitis at the age of three. She led them to his bed.

He was a thin, sad-looking young man, dark with a beaky nose, looking much older than his age. He smiled at the doctors, from under the great bandage that swathed his head. The doctors scarcely spoke to him, but addressed a few brief words to each other. Then one of them asked him to raise his left hand and touch his nose with it. With immense difficulty he lifted his arm, shaking a little, appearing to use only the muscles in his upper arm, the rest hanging limply. He got his hand to within three inches of his nose, but it stuck there, and he kept it there until the doctor told him to let it go. Then they hurried away again, with only a brief nod to the man.

The man being admitted had been kept waiting so long that he hadn't had anything to eat. So Anne hurried into the kitchen and found the most junior nurse, and asked her to make him some eggs on toast.

As she came out of the kitchen on the way to her desk to get the key for the egg cupboard another doctor stopped her and said, 'I've just seen Mr Hill. He seems to be wrapped in a great wad of paper and gauze. I thought he'd be more comfortable in a sanitary towel and a belt, and he said he didn't mind, so could you see to it?' She had to have the name and complaint of every one of her twenty-seven patients absolutely at her fingertips all the time. She went on to find the key.

On the way she passed a bed with the curtains drawn round, and she put her head inside. A man was lying with a huge square wad of cotton wool over his stomach, and three separate tubes (or drains) coming out of him. He looked mournful, and was snapping at the nurse tending to him. A label, 'Nil by mouth', was sellotaped to the bedstead. He swore to himself crossly. She said one or two firmly comforting words to him. She explained to me that he had been a very heavy drinker and tended to get confused without drink. He had had an enormous pancreatic abscess removed and was at times difficult and stubborn.

The little nurse came out of the kitchen to look for her. 'Have you got that key to the egg cupboard?' she asked. They went back to the kitchen and tried every key on her chain, but not one of them fitted the egg cupboard. An older nurse came along to help, but she couldn't make any of the keys fit either.

As Anne came out of the kitchen one of the student nurses came and told her that Mr Hatch was very worried because the two doctors who had just examined him had gone away without telling him what they were going to do next. So she hurried over to Mr Hatch's bed and said, 'They weren't coming here to treat you. One of them was just handing over to his second man and wanted to introduce you, so he knew who you were. Don't worry, they weren't making any decisions about you behind your back.' He smiled and said he was sorry to have bothered her. 'I'm sorry we didn't explain,' she said, smiling too.

An embarrassed priest was hovering round the desk when she came back. She led him to the patient he wanted to see.

She went back to the kitchen to see if any progress had been made on the egg cupboard, but none had. So she told the nurse to borrow some eggs from the next-door ward, and she went and told the ward clerk to get someone to come up and see to the door. 'We have to keep everything in the kitchen locked,' she said. 'People used to wander in off the street and help themselves before. It's part of being in this area of London where there are many people wandering around who are hungry. One day I caught a woman sitting in the kitchen eating a jam sandwich and actually drinking a cup of tea she had made for herself. She ran off when I asked her who she was.'

The evening newspaper seller was doing her round of the ward. It was time for Anne to check the consumption of controlled drugs administered in the last twenty-four hours against the amount supposed to be in stock. This was a long, complicated, boring and time-consuming business. But every single controlled (i.e. possibly addictive) drug had to be accounted for. She had never lost one yet, that could not be accounted for. She unlocked the large medicine cupboard, drew out the long register of drugs and proceeded to check each ampoule, count each pill, and the level of each bottle against what had been signed out. Just as she had taken them all out the telephone on the desk rang. No one answered it. She looked round to see if there was another nurse in sight, but there wasn't, so she had to bundle everything back into the cupboard, shut and padlock it and hurry over to the desk, by which time the telephone had stopped ringing. She went back to finish the drug check.

The telephone rang again, this time answered by Sister. She put it down and came up to Anne at the drug cupboard. 'Guess what? They've just phoned to say that Mr Pollard has had a barium enema, and now he has to have a rectal enema every three hours, poor chap. That's not very nice. By the way, are the little ones back from tea yet?' Anne said they would be in a minute.'

A doctor came to look at the new patient's perianal abscess. Afterwards a man from a few beds up, waiting for an operation on his haemorrhoids the next day came and sat beside him, and they were soon deep into discussion of the relative discomfort of their ailments.

Anne went into a side room to help with the setting up of a Vernon Thomson pump. This was to be attached to a drain the patient had emerging from his back. They had some trouble getting it right. The man had been stabbed in a fight and his lung had become infected and needed draining. 'I had one of those before,' he said out of the side of his mouth. He didn't take his eyes off the television which happened, aptly, to be showing *Police Surgeon*. When it was fixed Anne came out. She said, 'He can be very demanding. He's just waiting to get out and get his revenge. I've tried talking him out of it but he doesn't appreciate that two wrongs don't make a right.'

It was tea time. But Anne said she had to find time to talk to Mr Carter, the seventy-year-old who had had a serious intestinal operation for cancer, and now had a colostomy.

He was in a bed in the main ward by the door, lying propped up with a number of pillows, a tube emerging from his nose, and a drip attached to his arm. 'I'm so sad about him,' Anne said. 'Old people often get confused after they've had an operation. It seems to be harder for them to orientate themselves. He was fine yesterday, and I didn't think he would become confused. I talked to him a lot in the last few days.'

She approached his bed and asked how he was. He smiled at her and nodded. 'Shall I help you sit up a bit more?' she asked. He nodded again. She called over a student nurse and together they lifted him up and remade his bed for him. She talked to him the while and he nodded. He seemed to understand, until he began to talk himself, and then it was apparent that he was babbling, and didn't really know where he was. She patted the bed, and his hand, and went down to the Sister's room for tea, passing a small solid physiotherapist in brown stretch trousers and sneakers who was excercising the young man with meningitis.

In the Sister's room a few of the senior nurses from the next ward had congregated as well. The talk was mostly shop. Tea seemed to be over all too soon. It was interrupted three times by junior nurses asking for things, or bringing messages.

When it was time to get back to work there seemed to be even more to do. 'Did you remember that Mr Wells needs transport to Hammersmith for his neutron beam treatment?' one nurse was asking Anne anxiously.

'The man from Buxton Ward, Mr George, with a lipoma on his neck is going to theatres tomorrow morning, they rang to say,' reported another nurse.

'Ah,' said Anne. 'I haven't got to know him yet. He's only just arrived, hasn't he?'

Another nurse came up. 'Admissions say are we expecting to admit a Mr Sin Fan Tong today? He's waiting.'

Anne groaned quietly. 'Would you tell them we know nothing about him. We haven't got a bed. We have one patient waiting outside to be admitted already, and we aren't even sure if we can take him, until we hear from the consultant whether Mr Calthorpe can go home today.'

'What shall I say then?' asked the nurse anxiously.

'Say I'll call them as soon as I know about Mr Calthorpe.'

Anne brushed back one of the two stray wisps of hair that had fallen from under her cap. A woman with glasses came up to her and said 'I'm from CSSD. Have you finished your stock level sheets yet?'

'Goodness me, no!' Anne said, but smiled kindly at her. 'I'll let you have them as soon as they're done.' The CSSD is the Central Sterile Supplies Department, who are responsible for sterilizing and packing all the different packages of dressings, and providing all the disposable instruments.

It was four o'clock and already the ward seemed dark. The phone rang by the nurses' desk. 'Talbot Ward. Can I help you?' Anne said as she answered it. 'Yes, yes. He had his operation today, and he's quite comfortable. I'm afraid I can't discuss that over the telephone. Who is that speaking? I see. Well, no, no visiting today, better tomorrow. He's still a little drowsy. Visiting is between quarter to seven and eight. Thank you,' and she replaced the receiver.

She looked through her notes. In order to remember everything that people kept saying to her, she kept notes in a notebook in a pocket under her apron. She also, like all nurses, sometimes jotted down reminders on the inside corner of her apron. After a quick check in the book, she approached the new admission with the perianal abscess, who still appeared to be engrossed in vivid swapping of medical tales with another patient, and told him to have a bath, ready for his operation that evening. His was not a bad abscess, and didn't appear to be causing great pain. He would be out in a couple of days. She went to find him an operating gown and clean towel for his bath. She couldn't find a gown, and as she was searching a young nurse called her over quickly to Mr Carter in the next room.

Mr Carter, the elderly confused man, was lying back on his pillows staring at the ceiling. He had no drip in his arm now, nor a tube from his nose. 'He pulled them all out,' the nurse said. There was a dish of tubing on his table. The nose tube was long, as it had reached all the way down to his stomach. 'He got out of bed and I found him all over the place,' she said. 'Shall I put the nasal tube back?

'No, not for the moment,' said Anne. She went over to him and put a kindly hand on his arm. He gazed at her as if he didn't recognize her at all, though she'd often talked to him. 'Mr Carter, are you all right?' she asked. He didn't answer, so she left him. 'I hope they'll say he needn't have the tube,' she said. 'I think it upsets him too much. It would be worth letting him drink, even if it wasn't the normal medical treatment.'

Back at the desk a nurse was asking, 'Mr Calthorpe, is he going home?' Anne thought she had better try and find out if a decision had been made. Mr Calthorpe was waiting to go, a new patient was waiting outside to come in, but the doctor couldn't be found. Anne called again and this time she found him. Yes, Mr Calthorpe's tests were clear and he could go.

'Has he got an appointment card for out-patients?' Anne asked the nurse, who went off to find out. Anne asked another nurse to fit up cot sides to Mr Carter's bed, to stop him climbing out again.

The other nurse came back. 'He's got a card. What about his TTAs?' (TTA means 'To Take Away'.) Anne found his medicines, and took them to him to explain slowly and carefully exactly how many spoonfuls of each bottle he should have how many times a day.

At that moment Mr Rabkin, the one who'd been sent for a bath, put his head round the bathroom door, and blushing a little, called out to Anne if she'd found the towel and gown she was going to get him. She went to get them for him.

She stopped on the way to ask the hallucinator whether his pain was better after the increased dose, and he said it was much improved, but he could do with another dose perhaps. So she went to get it for him, bringing her bunch of keys out from under her apron to open the medicine trolley. As she unlocked it two doctors came in. 'Thank you, Staff,' said one politely. 'But could you tell me where we can find the boy who fell off his bike and fractured his mandible?' She relocked the trolley and led them to a bed in the next room.

Then she came back to the trolley, unlocked it again, and took out two tablets from a bottle. She called over a nurse to double-check that it was the right drug and dose, and then put the pills on a spoon on a little wicker tray that looked as if it had come from the occupational therapy department. She locked up the trolley and took the man his pills, went back to the trolley, and locked it to the pillar.

The man put his head out of the bathroom door again, and she handed him the towel and gown, and he blushed again.

It was time to go and oversee the work of the student nurse

who had been making the half-hourly observations on the patient with the fractured jaw. She went up to his bed and examined the plottings the nurse had made on a graph. 'It's not that I doubt their ability to make proper observations, but one has to make sure that the students know what they're looking for.' But everything was in order, so she hung his notes back on the end of the bed.

She stopped to help a nurse make the bed of the man in the bath, next door to the bed of the man who had hallucinations. At that moment several doctors, one an American that the Sister said looked just like Elliot Gould, came to see the hallucinator. They asked him what he'd been seeing.

'I saw you, actually,' he said with some embarrassment. 'I was talking to this nurse, and I kept seeing you out of the corner of my eye. When I turned to talk to you, you were never there.'

'But it's better now?' Anne asked him.

'It seems to be. But it was a very nasty experience, very upsetting,' he said.

The man came out of the bathroom and got into his newly made bed.

'You'll be having your pre-med soon,' Anne told him. 'It'll make you a bit drowsy before you go up to theatres.' Somehow it seemed odd for someone to be having an operation in the evening. It was quite dark outside now.

She apologized for not knowing exactly when his operation would be, but explained that towards the end of the lists the timings get harder to judge. 'I can promise you it'll be shortly, anyway,' she said to him. She sounded a bit like an air stewardess apologizing for a late take-off.

She went to help make another bed, before it was time for the pre-supper evening medicine round. These rounds took a long time, as it was an opportunity for the Sister or Staff Nurse to talk to each patient individually and see how they were feeling, or whether they seemed unduly depressed.

Anne and a young Chinese student nurse pushed round the

big medicine trolley together, starting at the first bed in the big room at the end of the corridor.

'Hello, Mr Phillips. How are you feeling?' This patient awoke with a start, and said he still had a head-ache. 'Had your bowels open today?'

'No, not for three days,' he answered sleepily. Anne poured him a little plastic medicine cup of a sticky, nasty-looking laxative. She wrote a note about his head-aches.

The man in the next bed was also asleep. 'Mr Weston!' Anne called. She had taken his chart from the end of the bed and was reading it. He jumped awake suddenly.

'What's the matter with you, then? Was I looking too happy for you, or something?' he said in a strong Welsh accent. He had a funny-looking gauze skull-cap on his head. He was a youngish man, in his early thirties, and he was a fast talker. 'I'd better have some of the white stuff too. . . . Aw, not that peppermint one, haven't you sold out of that yet?' Mr Weston was given his medicine and pills on the little wicker tray. He had recently had an acoustic neuroma removed, an ear operation.

As Anne pushed the trolley on to the next bed on the other side of the ward she explained to Nurse Tan and me that Mr Weston had been a rather quiet and different person before his operation. 'Brain surgery often makes people seem a bit tipsy for quite a long time afterwards. We don't get many neuro-surgery patients in this ward. He'll probably settle down in a few days.'

The next man was due for a major operation the next day, a hemi-colectomy, which might mean a colostomy. He seemed quite lively and not depressed when they asked him how he was. He said he was hot, but the diarrhoea was better.

As they moved on there began to be some terrible snorting noises, chokes and muffled protests from behind the closed curtains round poor Mr Carter's bed. A doctor and a nurse were putting the tube back down his throat. This meant the patient had to keep swallowing it until it reached the stomach. Anne was a little upset, and said again that she thought it would do more harm than good. She considered his total health, and thought he stood a better chance of making a good recovery if he could regain his spirits and full understanding. 'It'll set him back a lot I'm afraid,' she said. 'It'll frighten him.'

The next man was cheerful, though he had had a serious intestinal blockage and now had a colostomy. 'I wish I could eat something,' he said to Anne as she handed him his medicine. 'I'm only allowed to drink. I could just do with a steak and chips.'

She smiled and said, 'Well, perhaps you'll be able to have some one day.'

He sighed. 'Trouble is, by the time that day comes I won't be able to afford it, the way prices are going,' he said.

The next man was Mr Morley, the patient with a gangrenous toe, and iscaemic disease. He was tall and gaunt, and sat bolt upright in his bed, with a great wire cage over his foot, covered by the blankets. He looked austere and stern, with cavernous cheeks and fierce eyes, like a watchful eagle. From out of the controlled drug section of the medicine trolley, Anne drew a bottle, a plain, glass, medicine bottle with 'BRANDY' printed in bold black letters on the label. Next to it was another identical bottle with 'SHERRY' marked on it. They looked like Alice in Wonderland's 'Drink Me' bottle. Anne unscrewed the plastic top and poured a full medicine beaker of brandy, about the size of a pub double measure. 'He has this four times a day,' she said, as she placed it on the little tray. 'Brandy is good for the veins. It dilates them and helps the circulation. Also he's a little depressed.' She took out a large black and red capsule and put it on a spoon for him, and took him the tray. He nodded, but didn't smile, sipped the drink with the pill, and put the rest beside his bed, and they moved on. I asked if the other patients knew that brandy could be prescribed, and whether they didn't ask for it too? She said they didn't.

The young man with his head bandaged was sitting in a chair by his bed. He said he still had some facial pain, so he was given something for it, and some white laxative.

133

In the end bed was a patient who had been in the ward for a long time, several months, a man all the nurses knew well. Anne gave him his pills, and as she was stepping away he caught her hand and started talking rapidly, quietly. Then he suddenly broke into sobs, and she sat beside him for a little, and pulled the curtain half way along his bed. 'But you're getting so much better,' she was saying. 'Remember what you were like three weeks ago, and think how much better you'll be in three weeks' time.' The man had had a bowel operation with many complications.

'I was fourteen stone when I came in here,' he was saying. 'Now look at me!' He was tiny and thin. Eventually he cheered up a bit, and then suddenly became quite jolly.

Lying neatly on the next bed was an elegant middle-aged man, in beautifully pressed yellow pyjamas and a subtle shaded paisley dressing-gown, ending in crisp leather slippers. They decided to let him sleep, as he had been taken off all painkillers and was allowed no food until the morning when he was to have some special blood tests.

In the last bed in the big room was Mr Carter. The curtains had been drawn back from his bed now, and he was lying on his pillows, looking a little dazed, the tube from his nose to his stomach back in place, the drip plugged back into his arm. Anne shook her head sadly. She pulled on a pair of surgical gloves, took out a disposable syringe, and three different ampoules of fluid. These she showed to Nurse Tan to check for accuracy, before breaking them open, dipping in the needle and drawing the stuff into the syringe. She told Mr Carter loudly that he was going to have a small injection, and it wouldn't hurt. He rolled his head toward her on the pillow and nodded, with an attempt at a smile. She injected the drugs into his vein, in the hole where the drip was, as this was less painful, and he didn't appear to notice. He picked up a copy of *Reader's Digest* from his bed, perched his spectacles on top of the nose tube and started to read, but he put it down again, as if the effort was too much.

They were wheeling the trolley into the other part of the

ward when Mr Weston, the Welshman who had had an ear operation called out, 'I think I'll jump out of this bed in the nude and scream. Oh, then you'd laugh!' and Anne smiled at him and moved on.

'He's definitely a bit tipsy,' Anne said. However Mr Morley, who had had the brandy, did not look in the least tipsy. The cup was empty, and he was still sitting there, the gaunt eagle look in his eye.

In the other part of the ward, which divided into three sections of four beds, a man with a stick and a hospital green candlewick dressing-gown was sitting on a chair. When he was asked what he wanted he sang out, 'Milpar, Umpah, Stick it up your jumper!' so they laughed kindly and poured him some of the sickly white laxative. He prodded the Chinese nurse with his stick and said, 'You don't understand English, do you?' but she took it in good part.

The man with the fractured jaw, whose teeth had been wired together and was under half-hourly observation, was given an injection in his behind. It was an antibiotic, and stuff to stop him vomiting, which was a danger to patients who couldn't open their mouths. He groaned loudly and they told him to roll onto his side. As Anne jabbed the needle into him, not unlike throwing a dart, she told him to wiggle his toes. Then they lifted him up on the pillows and smoothed his covers.

The next patient, the young man waiting for a haemorrhoid operation the next day, needed nothing. 'What's this then, nurse,' he asked, pointing at me with my notebook. 'Time and motion?'

Sister started to bring round the soup trolley for supper for those too ill to get out of bed. There were only another three patients left for the medicine round, and the smell of soup filled the air.

Once the medicine trolley was locked away Sister came up and asked Anne, 'Is Mr Rabkin pre-meded for theatres yet?'

'No,' Anne said. 'Do we know yet when he's going?'

Sister called up to theatres to ask them how they were doing, and when to expect Mr Rabkin to be called for his perianal abscess operation. They said they'd call back.

Sister asked Anne if she would mind writing the Matron's Report. She referred to her as Matron, although now Matrons are known as Nursing Officers. The report had to be sent every evening listing all newly admitted patients – after most of which 'Has settled well' would be written – and all seriously ill patients, of whom there were none at the moment. (Seriously ill in this case means in imminent danger of death.) Patients prepared for operation, and their condition after operation were also reported.

There then followed an interchange with the Admissions office, and it was determined that following the unexpected sending home of one patient, there would after all be room for Mr Sin Fan Tong, a sixteen-year-old who had been waiting downstairs to be admitted for an ear operation. He was duly sent up, arrived at the ward, and was admitted by one of the juniors to the empty bed next to Mr Carter. He was a pretty boy who scarcely spoke. 'Mr Sin Fan Tong has settled well,' Anne wrote on her Matron's Report.

These reports are kept for five years, and can be used as legal documents. They are intended to keep Matron informed of the main events in each ward each day.

The phone rang on the desk. It was theatres saying not to expect Mr Rabkin's operation for at least another hour. Anne decided to give him his pre-med. Theatres said a Mr Malloney has just gone in. Unfortunately they'd been too late with him to give him a pre-med at all.

It was now 6.45 and supper was long over. A gathering crowd had been assembling at the door of the ward for the last twenty minutes. An assortment of people of all ages and sizes, wearing outdoor coats, looking oddly out of place amongst the white sheets and uniforms, carrying pots and bunches of flowers, brown bags of fruit, most of it probably bought at the keen and thrusting stalls outside the hospital in the Whitechapel Road. Sister let them in and they broke into

136

the ward, almost at the trot, like ladies who have queued all night outside a department store sale. They spread themselves around the various beds. The telephone started to ring. 'Talbot Ward, can I help you?' Anne said into it. 'Yes, yes, yes, I see. Point three seven nought? Thank you. I'll tell doctor.' It was a blood result from the clinical laboratories and she added it to the patients' lists.

Two old men were standing, hats in hands, waiting politely for her to finish on the telephone, and Anne turned to them. 'Mr Goldstein, if you please?' one of them asked politely in a strong foreign accent.

She got to her feet and smiled and shook her head. 'I'm very sorry, but Mr Goldstein has left us. He is not with us any more,' she said slowly as their English didn't appear to be good.

'Gone?' asked one incredulously, and she saw that for a moment they might have thought she meant dead.

'Yes, to the country,' she added quickly. 'To a convalescent home, to get better. To Banstead.'

'Is that far?' one of them asked.

'Yes,' she answered. 'A long way, I'm afraid. I'm sorry you've had all the trouble of coming up here.' The two men bowed and departed.

Then Sister announced that it was supper time, so she and Anne left and made their way to the Sisters' dining-room, which is used by Staff Nurses as well, and also by a number of the administrative staff. Dining-rooms in the hospital are rigidly segregated. The consultants have their own, with waiters, the doctors another. There was this one for Sisters, and another for juniors and a fifth canteen for the remainder. Some democrats in the hospital were trying to get this all changed, but there was great opposition.

When Anne came back from her half-hour supper break, there were still two more hours of hard work ahead of her before handing over to the night staff at ten o'clock. She wrote reports, did another drug round, checked the CSSD supplies, gave the student nurses a teaching session, went round with one or two doctors who had a quick last look at their patients, and finally settled the patients down for the night.

By the time she left she was quite exhausted. She did not have a particularly strong physique, and often got too tired. She had managed to arrange now that some of her days off should be interspersed with her working days, to give herself a rest, instead of having to wait ten or eleven days before getting all her rest days together in a lump.

Anne lived in the nurses' home, a modern and luxurious block at the back of the hospital where she shared a four-room flat with three other nurses, for about £20 a month. She liked living in, enjoying the companionship. But some nurses commute some distance, which must be tiring after a long late shift.

As she had to be back on duty at eight the next morning, she had little time that night to do more than sleep. 'I find it difficult sometimes to unwind,' she said. 'I get so tired that my mind keeps going at such a pace – all the things to do and to remember. I find sometimes I can't sleep for a long time, and even then not well.'

In the morning, arriving back in the ward, it seemed such a short time since she had left it. She sat with her notebook, and I with mine and the night Staff Nurse gave her report. Some of the youngest juniors looked quite tired and bleary-eyed. The night, it seemed, had been uneventful. No admissions, no dramas. One or two patients had slept badly and had fretfully paced the ward. Mr Carter had pulled out his tube and drip twice more, and was now waiting for a decision from the doctors about what should be done next.

After the report was over came the medicine round. By now the patients had been up for a long time, and breakfast was long ago. Some were back dozing on their beds. This round took even longer, and was conducted by Sister as well as Anne. They were carefully inspecting their charges, to see how they were, compared with the night before. 'You must stay in bed, my love,' Sister said gently to Mr Carter as they passed his bed at the start of the round.

Mr Philips complained again of head-aches, 'A real cracker this morning,' he said. Mr Morley had another large brandy, which seemed less appealing at this hour of the day.

Mr Weston, the 'tipsy' one, came hurrying back to his bed as they approached it, smelling powerfully of scent. 'Don't you ever wash, just dab on some after-shave?' Sister teased. 'What is it, Hi Karate or something?'

'Hi Karate?' he expostulated. 'I wouldn't insult my body with that stuff. It's Eau de Sauvage,' he said, twisting his lips elaborately round the French words.

The next man was given castor oil. He was due for an operation that day. Mr Carter clattered something to the ground, and Anne went back to pick it up for him before proceeding. 'There's only two kinds of medicine in this ward,' grumbled the next patient. 'One to make you go and one to stop you.' The young man with a bandaged head was given liquid paraffin. Then there was the man who had wept the evening before. Anne had hardly given him his pills and medicine before he started to weep again. He told her of his great wrestling feats when he was young. Then he wept some more and told her, between sobs, that he had accidentally killed his best friend at judo and could never forget it, and he felt so guilty. She asked him when it had happened, and he said it was in 1940. He wiped away his tears, swigged his medicine and said the trouble was, he hadn't had much sleep the night before. His scar was leaking a bit and he was worried this would set him back and he wouldn't get out so soon. She reassured him.

The perfect yellow pyjamas still looked as if they had just been ironed. Perhaps they were a different pair. He was white and drawn this morning, and winced when spoken to. He said the pain was bad, and asked if he couldn't have just a little something for it? Anne apologized with great sincerity but said he must wait till he had the blood tests; it shouldn't be too long now.

The young Chinese boy would go for his ear operation

today. He didn't need medicine. One of the consultant's registrars came in. 'Good morning Sister, good morning Staff,' he said, almost with a click of the heels. 'Any catastrophes this morning? No? Good.' He went to look at one or two special patients. At the same time a small team of neuro-surgeons arrived to see one of their patients.

Mr Carter came next. He smiled and touched Anne's hand when she came up to him to ask how he was. She and Sister pulled back his bedclothes to straighten them. His pyjamas and bedclothes had watery blood stains on them. When Anne pulled up his pyjama top to look at his stitches and colostomy, she saw he had been pulling at them. He had pulled his colos-tomy bag half off, though there was nothing much in it since he hadn't eaten for a week. She straightened him out, and a little later told one of the other nurses to change his bed. 'I hope they'll let him drink this morning', she said. 'I can't see it would harm him. He'd feel a lot better!' She jotted a note about him down in her book. Then they gave him another injection. Again, Anne protected her hands with surgical gloves. This is to stop nurses, who handle so many antibiotics, from developing a reaction to it themselves.

A doctor came past and Anne managed to ask him if he would change his mind about keeping that patient in yellow pyjamas off all painkillers until he'd had a blood test. The doctor looked at the man, saw he was suffering, and relented. Anne returned and gave him an injection.

At the other side of the ward some young nurses came up to Mr Cotton, the austere-looking man who was prescribed brandy. One of them was carrying a large bowl of warm water. 'Mr Cotton, wake up! Wake up!' one of them said, putting a hand on his shoulder and shaking him a little. 'We're going to give you a wash.'

He awoke and said sharply, 'You just set down that bowl here, and I'll do it myself, thank you.'

They agreed. 'All right, we'll leave you with everything you need,' and they pulled the curtains round him.

Mr Rabkin, the man who had had his abscess operated on the

previous evening, came slowly up to Anne to ask if he could have a bath. She left the trolley with Sister and took him to the bathroom to show him the salt he should add to the water.

Then another doctor called her away to ask her about an admission there had been to another ward late last night of a man who had once been in Talbot. She remembered the man's name at once, even though he had only stayed in Talbot one night, and that was over a month ago. Her memory was almost phenomenal. She checked with the doctor in the admissions book. Then the telephone rang. While she answered it, the Chinese boy was wheeled away by a porter for X-rays. 'Mr Simpson? Yes. And also Mr Phillips, please,' she was saying.

Mr Simpson's bed was not far from the telephone. He called out, 'Me? Is it for me? I'm Mr Simpson!'

She replaced the receiver and went over to him. 'No, Mr Simpson, it wasn't for you. It was just about some tests you had.'

'Oh,' he said, looking disappointed. 'I thought it might be my son calling from Australia to see how I was. He called last week, and it cost him £50!'

Two old men sitting on a bed next to him were discussing some people they both knew. This is still enough of a community hospital for several patients in this ward to have known each other a little, and to have friends and acquaintances in common from the East End. 'I live down the No Entry street by the Whitbread's pub, opposite the pie shop,' one said.

'Oh, I go in that pie shop all the time. Wish I was there now!' said the other.

Sister and another nurse had reached the man with the wired-together jaw. He looked much better, was sitting up in bed, sucking orange juice through a straw. The next man was given castor oil that he mixed with a lot of undiluted lemon squash, which must have made it taste even worse. A very small Swiss man in the next bed who had only been in three days for a dental operation was due to leave. He was sitting on the bed, with a bald head and gold glasses, putting his shoes on. He looked like a small leprechaun. Anne said, when we had passed him, 'The social worker found that he lives alone without electricity, poor man. But he seems very happy and is determined to go home today.'

After a couple more patients with colostomies, the round was eventually over. I asked Anne if she could imagine having a colostomy herself. 'No,' she said. 'I wouldn't like to have one.' She paused to think about it. 'Well, it's really a matter of determination, determination to carry on and manage, I suppose.'

An older nurse had joined us, and she said, 'Well, an awful lot of well-known people have them, and you'd never guess.'

Mr Carter called Anne over again. 'Is the barber coming today?' he asked. She said she'd send the barber to shave him as soon as he came. She went to chain the medicine trolley back to its pillar.

She asked two of the nurses to go and do some of the dressings. Almost all dressings were changed once a day, in the mornings. She herself then went to do two of the more complicated ones taking one of the students with her to explain why and show her how. Then the barber arrived – a small dapper man with elegantly cut white hair, and a bad limp in one leg. He had worked in the hospital for years, and was a favourite with the nurses. He carried a big wooden box over his shoulder, and the pockets of his white overall were bursting with scissors and combs. Anne stopped him and asked him to shave Mr Carter, to cut Mr Morley's hair, and to shave another patient's stomach.

She then gave a pre-med to one of yesterday's new admissions who was waiting for an operation, and called through to theatres to try to get some idea when to pre-med the others who were being operated on that day.

At last, it was lunch time. Anne and Sister hurried away for a brief half-hour in the Sisters' dining-room. I had the chance over lunch to ask her a little more about herself. There was never any time on the ward for anything more than the briefest explanations of what was going on.

She is a devout Christian, and belongs to the Nurses' Christian Fellowship, which has regular meetings. Her family live in Essex, and she is one of five children. Her father commuted to London and worked for the Central Electricity Generating Board. She has an older sister who is a teacher, and younger sister who veers between wanting to teach and wanting to nurse. One brother works for an engineering firm, and the other, her twin, is a chartered accountant. Her father hadn't wanted her to take up nursing. He was appalled by the idea. But once she had set her mind on it, and had been accepted by the local general hospital, it was he who found out about the teaching hospitals and encouraged her to try for The London, despite her apparent lack of qualifications.

She plays tennis and swims in the hospital pool, and sometimes goes to the Feathers Club, a nurses' club for hospital staff and medical students. There are numerous clubs and societies run by the medical students which the nurses are encouraged to join, but she always finds that she can't attend them regularly due to working shifts.

She remembered how frightened she was when she first started nursing. 'You've had only eight weeks' teaching when you start on a ward. It's quite terrifying. In a way I was lucky as the first ward I was given was in the private wing, where there were only twelve patients. But I made a mistake. I can't think how I did it. The tutors say there's always one fool who does it. I sat a patient down on a commode, having forgotten to put a bed pan in it.'

She was cautious in what she said about the role of nurses. 'Some of the older consultants treat the nurses as if they were servants, and yet some of them are most polite. It varies.' She said she saw nurses as intermediaries between doctors and patients. 'Often a patient is overcome by awe on the doctors' rounds, and he will say, "I'm fine, thank you, doctor," when you know quite well he's been in a lot of pain, and isn't well. You have to tell doctors these things. How are they to know, when perhaps they don't see the patient for more than a few minutes a day? The patients get scared by things they think the doctors have said, or things they haven't understood. You have to act as interpreter, both ways, between doctors and patients. Also, we like to try and soften the blow, if we can. If a doctor lets us know what he's about to tell a patient, if it's something bad, we like to try and prepare him for the possibilities gently, so it doesn't come as a complete shock on the ward round, with all those bewildering doctors and students there.'

She found her last post, where she was caring for leukaemic patients, some of whom were young, a great strain. 'I was on that ward for nine months, and by the time I was leaving many of the patients I had nursed when they were first diagnosed were dying. By then I knew them very well indeed, as they would come into the ward regularly for treatment and I found it hard to bear. In some ways though, it was nice, because I did know them so well, that I really could comfort them. How do you comfort someone who is dying? Well, all you can do is listen when they want to talk, show you care. If they ask me for my views I would gladly tell them, or if it came up in conversation. But as a nurse it is very important not to misuse your position by forcing your views on other people. No, it hasn't made me afraid of dying.' She thought for a moment before saying, 'My first death was the worst, in a way, although the patient wasn't young. He was an old man, very sweet. He had nothing and no one in the whole world, not a single friend or relative, and that seemed terrible to me. When he died all there was left was an old shirt, and I cried. Dying alone is sad, but I have no fear of death because of the faith that I have.'

As we came back from lunch the phone was ringing on the desk. Anne picked it up. 'No, no, Mrs Simon, it's really nothing at all, nothing to worry about. . . . Let me explain. . . . No. . . .

Look. . . .' she sighed as she didn't have a chance to get a word in to explain. 'There is nothing to worry about, Mrs Simon,' she said. 'He is not having another operation. The reason we didn't let him eat or drink last night or this morning, and we took him off all drugs is just that he has to have some blood tests this morning, routine blood tests, which eating might effect. Yes. That's all right. Thank you. That's quite all right. Good-bye.' She replaced the receiver and called over a young nurse. 'Has Sin Fan Tong had a bath yet? Could you see he does, please?' she said.

Sister was looking towards Mr Shona, the patient who had a fractured jaw, and who yesterday had seemed so ill. 'Have you noticed how the Indian patients seem to sleep all day in hospital? Isn't it strange?' she said. 'Oughtn't we to get him up for a bit?'

There was now an anxious atmosphere of anticipation building up in the ward. One of the consultants was about to come on his weekly ward round, and he was a man they were all nervous of. He was one of the consultants that treated nurses harshly, often found fault, made them feel awkward and stupid, and rarely asked their opinion. Anne and Sister both felt apprehensive.

'I don't think he has any idea at all how much work we do, or what it's like to run a busy ward all day long. If the consultants could spend a day on a ward, they could perhaps understand what it's like, and what it's reasonable to expect,' Anne said.

Both nurses were agreed that this man was not the worst. There were other consultants, whom they considered even more unpleasant to the nurses. This wasn't the way Sister and Anne viewed all consultants. They both said that many were very charming, and helpful.

The man who had been stabbed came down the corridor, the drain from his back leading down to a flagon which he carried in one hand. He had a number of clamps sticking out of his bandages and dressing-gown. He made his way slowly to the telephone trolley, and wheeled it back to his room.

One old man, a great talker, had cornered his favourite student nurse for the fifth time that day and was telling her some long story, to which she listened politely before extricating herself as soon as she could, saying, 'Well! You have had an interesting life, Mr Evans!' as if it were all over already.

Anne decided to give Sin Fan Tong his pre-med, as she saw the boy emerge from the bathroom and make his way back to bed. She went to the medicine trolley and looked up the amount of drugs the anaesthetist had prescribed. She groaned when she saw it. It was an odd dosage, with 70 mg., instead of the normal 75 of one drug, and 30 instead of 35 of the other. Since the ampoules came in standard sizes, it was very hard to calculate. She thought about it, and then rang the doctor to ask him if he had really meant it, as it was a very hard dose to administer accurately. He said yes, he meant it. She was a little annoyed, since she knew it made practically no difference at all whether he had 5 mg. over or under. 'The doctors often don't realize what amounts these drugs come in. They calculate the amount needed by the patient's bodyweight, but it would be easier if they kept it to the nearest easily dividable part of a hundred.' Sister came over to help. Anne got out her notebook and tried to work out how to get the dose right.

Mr Hatch, the meningitis victim, came slowly up to the trolley. 'Can you tell me when I'm to go to the gym?' he asked quietly. 'I think they've missed me out today, and the physiotherapist did say I was to go.' Anne said she'd find out about it, and she wrote a note in her book, and went back to her calculations. 'I do think I *need* to go,' Mr Hatch said, and she was surprised that he was still standing there. 'My arm feels, well odd.'

'As if it wasn't a part of you?' Anne asked.

'Yes, that's it,' he said.

'But you're doing *so* well,' she said smiling at him. 'It used to be all tense, do you remember?'

'Sometimes I can't feel it.'

'Well, you must just keep remembering how it was, and how much better it's getting all the time,' she said. And he looked pleased and went back to his bed.

'So, we want a fifth of two-tenths of one ampoule, and two-tenths of the other, see?' she said to Sister.

'Oh dear, I never even got a CSE in maths,' Sister said. They put their heads together again and went over all the workings to see that they both understood. Just then a young doctor came up.

'Hello,' he said. He had a nervous look. 'I wonder if we could move the pump on Mr Hill from the B to the A drain?'

Sister looked up and smiled. 'Why don't you do it yourself?' she asked and laughed.

The doctor looked a little flustered and said, 'Yes, OK, if you like,' and started to move away.

She caught his arm and laughed again, 'No, come on, I was only joking of course. I'll do it myself in just a moment.' The young man looked even more confused, blushed just a little, and went away smiling. The two nurses laughed. That doctor was in and out of the ward all the time, and as he was nervous he was often teased, though they liked him.

Finally, without further interruption, they got the dose right. Although neither of them thought it mattered all that much about absolute accuracy, they made certain every time that it *was* completely accurate, and that each was satisfied that this was so, since legally, if anything went wrong with the aneasthetic during the operation, they could be liable if they had mis-administered a dose by even a fraction.

The phone rang just as they had filled the syringe. It was theatres. Sister hurried back to Anne. 'We'd better hurry. They've just taken in a Mr Fawcett, and he's only having a biopsy, so Sin Fan Tong will be going up soon.'

They approached the boy's bed and drew the curtains round. They asked him if he wore false teeth or glass eyes, and he shook his head. They told him he was going to have his operation soon.

'Here?' he asked. They said no, upstairs. They asked him to

turn over so they could give him an injection in his behind. He seemed most reluctant.

'After you've had this you'll feel drowsy, and your mouth will feel dry. Please don't try to get out of bed, but press this bell for a nurse if you want anything.' He was wearing a hospital gown, after his bath. They pulled down the bed-clothes and tried to persuade him to roll over. But he held on to the bedclothes and looked worried. As there was some urgency about getting it done, Anne hurried away to find the Chinese Nurse Tan, as she thought perhaps the patient didn't understand what was happening to him. He looked particu-larly young, lying there anxiously, more like twelve than sixteen. Nurse Tan hurried along and translated rapidly.

The boy said with a perfect English accent, 'I know, I know, I understood everything,' and smiled. Finally he did roll over, and it turned out he was still wearing underpants which he was very shy about removing. The needle was jabbed into him, but it must have been skilfully done, since he didn't even wince, despite his nerves. He was also wearing a vest under his gown, which had to be taken off.

'Look, you just rest now,' Anne said to him. 'Nurse Tan will be going with you up to the theatres, so she'll be there.' It seemed a curious assumption that their common race would neccessarily comfort him, but he nodded and closed his eyes. A nurse from the ward goes up to the theatres with each patient, and stays until they are totally unconscious. They are then called back when the patient comes round in the recovery room and they accompany them back to the ward.

Mr Carter had been got out of bed, and now he was sitting in his chair he seemed much less ill than before. A nurse had wrapped his heels in large woolly pieces of sheep-skin, as his heels were in danger of developing pressure sores.

Anne stopped beside him to ask how he was. The doctors had not put up a drip or replaced the nose tube which he again pulled out that morning; he was still confused. 'How is the pain? Where is it?' Anne asked.

'Where?' he said. He got to his feet and started to look around for something. 'Where is what?' he asked.

'No, your pain, where do you feel it?' she said.

'Oh, all over my stomach.'

She told him the doctor would be round soon, and she would tell him about it.

Back at the desk a nurse was holding the telephone in one hand. She asked Anne, 'Who ordered the transport for that patient to go to Hammersmith hospital today?' Anne said the porters had, or should have, as she'd spoken to them about it this morning.

'Right, kids,' Sister said. 'Report time!' The new shift, the one-thirty shift, were coming on duty. The two shifts overlapped by one and a half hours. Sister read out the reports from the Kardex, and the new nurses took notes. When it was over the new Staff Nurse instructed her team of nurses, and the group disbanded.

'He's coming in a minute,' one of the nurses announced. 'He's just in the next ward.'

'Oh, God,' someone else said.

'I think I'll go in the loo and stay there,' Sister said.

'I always blush and feel guilty about everything he says,' Anne said.

She got out her notebook, and checked a list of current patients on a wall chart, jotting down the names of those who were under this consultant. She then telephoned the diet kitchen to order a high-protein fluid diet for the broken jaw patient. Just then a patient in a gown moved slowly towards the lavatory, and all at once three nurses rushed up to him and started ushering him back to bed, thinking he had already had a pre-med, ready for an operation, but it turned out he hadn't yet.

Then the great man arrived. He swept into the end of the ward, with his big entourage of young doctors hovering anxiously, wanting to hear what he said, but not wanting to get in the way, or attract his attention if they could help it.

Before there was time for Sister to explain who I was, he had gone into one of the side rooms, Sister and Anne accompanying him, well to the rear. When they all came out he led them for a moment into the patients' dining-room to discuss the case. Sister kept trying to interrupt, to find the right moment to explain who I was, but he spoke in a continuous flow that seemed impossible to break into. Finally, with great courage, and a little coughing, she managed. 'This is Polly Toynbee, who is with us on this ward this week. She is writing a book about the hospital. She is following Staff Nurse around. Miss Culpeck [the Divisional Nursing Officer] has arranged it. Would you mind if she came with Staff Nurse on your ward round?' she said in a rush, and blushed a little.

He stared at her, and then at me in a severe way, and left a dramatic silence, which I clumsily fell into.

'I've been in and out of the hospital for a year, and have been on a great many ward rounds. I hope you won't mind?' I asked.

He kept his silence before demanding, 'Are you a doctor?' I said I wasn't. I was a journalist. His eyebrows raised themselves. 'Well,' he said. 'You'd better pretend to be a doctor. I shall pretend to think you are.' And he moved off rapidly towards the main part of the ward. Sister breathed out with relief, and Anne and I stayed in the rear.

At the next patient's bed the consultant asked which doctor was to present the case. An embarassed young man came forward and started on the case history. The consultant interrupted him. 'Doctor, you're slipping from your good habits,' and he corrected the young man on the order of the facts he was presenting. They discussed the three tubes that protruded from this patient's abdomen, two of which were not draining anything, the third of which had just had a pump attached to it. He said the man was not to be given barium, but a special dye for his X-rays. He felt the man's stomach and said, 'Feel how rapidly this cavity is shrinking.' Some of the others had a feel. Before moving on he addressed the patient in a jocular fashion. 'Well, when we opened you up we found an abscess the size of your head, so there's a big cavity there now, but it's shrinking well.'

The man stared at him and blanched a little. 'The size of my head?' he asked incredulously.

The consultant answered, 'Or the size of mine, which is even bigger!' and they all moved on.

They passed a patient being taken away on a trolley to the operating theatre and came to Mr Carter, who was still sitting in a chair, looking deceptively spry. Anne pushed herself forward, as she had great concern for this man, wanted him not to have the nasal tube replaced and was worried about him being so confused. After some discussion with the doctors, the consultant turned to Mr Carter and asked him how he was. He complained of a lot of pain. 'You are bound to get that after a big operation like you've had,' said the consultant.

'Oh, it was a big operation then?' said Mr Carter.

'Yes indeed,' said the consultant, and turned to discuss the problems of the case.

Anne plucked up courage, as he was moving away, to say in a small voice, 'I'm afraid he's very confused at the moment.'

The consultant turned and looked at her and then laughed, 'I get that way myself!' he said. And they proceeded to the next bed.

His next patient was the man who had wept twice in the last two days on Anne's ward round. 'Ah, Mr Wilfer. You are my surgical triumph!' he said.

The man smiled back and then began to talk nervously. 'I've had a lot of pain, doctor. Last night I pulled at the big stitch. And now it's leaking again and I'm afraid it'll set me back. I worry about the pain, and the leaking.'

The consultant reminded him that he had told him to expect it to leak from time to time. He came away from the bed and shook his head. 'That man had seven operations before he came here. He's not doing badly.'

Mr Wilfer called him back, with a croak in his voice. 'January 7th, doctor, I'm booked on a holiday to Majorca.

I've got to pay the last instalment on it this week. Would you think that safe to do?'

The consultant smiled at him and said, 'I should think so, most probably. I'd bet on it, if I were a betting man.'

He had only four patients in the ward at the time. The last man was Mr Morley, the patient with gangrene who was being prescribed brandy. The poor man could probably have done with a good dose before suffering the shock he was about to get from the consultant.

The curtains were drawn round his bed, and all the doctors, the two nurses and I gathered round. The consultant rolled back the bedclothes from Mr Morley's legs. His foot was unbandaged, and rested under a wire cage that kept the weight of the covers off it. They discussed his case, which was presented by a different doctor. 'So you would suggest conservative management for the moment?' the consultant asked the young doctor. He said he would, and the consultant agreed. They discussed whether the gangrene was caused by a local embolism, or a more serious cut-off to the blood supply higher up his leg. The man also had a very bad leg ulcer on the back of his calf, which, they all agreed, almost certainly pointed to a lack of blood supply to the whole lower leg.

The foot, the big toe in particular, was dark red and black, though not suppurating. They all examined it. 'I'd say that was arterial all right,' the consultant said. Then, finally, he turned and spoke to the patient himself, who was still sitting bolt upright, his harsh bird-like look unchanged.

'Do you feel any pain?' asked the consultant. Mr Morley said he didn't. 'He's not diabetic, is he?' asked the consultant, turning to one of the doctors, who said he wasn't. 'Well, Mr Morley. I'm afraid this is a pretty serious situation,' he said. 'You have a case of dry gangrene. I have to tell you that there is a chance, quite a big chance, that we may have to take that bit of your leg off.'

The patient stared at him. 'Where from?' he asked. He was looking down at his own leg as if already it no longer belonged to him.

'From there, I think,' said the consultant, pointing to just above the knee.

'Couldn't you just take the toe off? I was expecting that,' Mr Morley asked.

The consultant said, 'Well, at present that's what we're hoping, of course. But we think the blood has been cut off higher up your leg, and if we operate just on the toe it wouldn't heal. That nasty ulcer of yours isn't healing at all. If we operate too low down we might have to do a second and a third operation, which would not be a good thing. I must in all frankness tell you that I think it likely it will end in amputation. If that toe on its own is enough, it'll probably separate itself soon. So we must wait and see.'

The man looked the consultant straight in the eye and said, 'I'm much obliged, doctor. I quite understand.' But then suddenly his face crumbled and turned from grey to pink. He pulled out a handkerchief and blew his nose loudly, but it didn't hide a great sob. The consultant turned and hurried away, followed by his entourage, anxious to beat a rapid retreat. Anne stayed and held his hand as he wept. It was particularly sad to see this great gaunt figure reduced to tears.

'Did you understand what the doctor was saying?' Anne asked him gently. 'If he just takes the toe off it won't heal and then you'll be in a worse state than you are now.'

'I wish he'd just take the toe off. I was prepared for that,' he said. The effort of talking drew him out of the tears, and he mopped his eyes and started to recover.

'They'll come and talk to you again about it, and of course, you know it's your own decision, don't you? If you say no, then they won't do it.'

'I know that. Yes, it's my decision. To tell the truth it's what I've been dreading to hear all the time I've been lying here.'

'You wouldn't be limited very much. In fact, with an artificial limb you'll get along a lot easier than you have on that leg for years now. A friend of mine lost his leg in a road accident and he's walking very well now with an artificial limb.'

'I expect that's true. It hasn't been good. It could be worse.' He blew his nose again. 'I suppose there's a lot of people worse off than me?'

'It would be the right thing to have done, if the doctor advises it.'

'You all understand a lot more about it than what I do.'

'Look on the bright side. You'll be a lot more mobile than you are now.'

'I'm so chicken-hearted, that's what I am,' he said, sufficiently recovered to be embarrassed by his tears.

'We all are. Don't worry,' she answered.

'If it's got to go, it's got to go.'

'What do you think your wife will think?' Anne asked gently.

'I'll have to tell her tonight,' he said. 'These people don't say these things for a joke, I suppose? I'll tell her.'

Anne reached across to his bedside table where a cup of tea was standing. 'Would you like to drink this, or is it too cold? I'll fetch you another if you like.'

He sipped it and said, 'It's fine. I don't like it too hot.'

She tucked the blankets round him. 'If you have any worries at all, just tell us,' she said. 'I'll come and chat to you a bit later myself. We'll always explain anything you want. Just remember that we've got some of the very best doctors in this hospital.'

He smiled, looked much better and said, 'I know that, and my wife knows that too.'

She drew back the curtains, smiled at him, and went back to the desk. When I asked her she said she thought the news had come to poor Mr Morley rather abruptly, and if she'd known that was what the consultant would say, she would have prepared the patient more gently for the shock. The consultant and his team had left the ward, and the atmosphere was more relaxed.

The barber came in and, seeing how busy she was, he joked to Anne, 'Staff, can you spare four hours of your time?' She laughed and told him which patients needed shaves and hair-cuts. She was still thinking about Mr Morley, and she turned to me and said, 'But you must realize that something like that isn't a blow you can soften very much. It doesn't make much difference how you say it, the fact itself is such a shock.'

The small Swiss patient who looked like a leprechaun was now about to leave. He was wearing a striped shirt of thick cotton, and a pair of trousers pulled up to his ribs with braces. He always smiled, and was immensely polite. He went round the ward, carrying a few things rolled in a newspaper and addressed each nurse, 'Your good health! You have been most kind, most kind. Thank you very much, so good of you, so kind,' he said to them all. Then he made his way out of the ward and down the corridor, leaving behind the slippers and pyjamas that belonged to the hospital. He had refused any help from the social workers who had discovered that he lived without even electricity.

Anne filled in a requisition form for a new electric light bulb. She told one of the nurses to change a dressing. As she walked past Mr Carter, who was drowsing in his chair, there was the loud sound of a fart from his colostomy bag. The poor man awoke with a jump, and she smiled at him. He went back to sleep.

A doctor came in and asked Anne if she could find out where his teaching session was supposed to be, as he'd been told it was in the lecture room at the end of the ward, but there was no one there.

She helped a nurse to make three beds, and then checked the pump on one patient's drain. He said he didn't think Staff Nurses made beds, which made her indignant, since she made dozens of beds a day, every day. 'He's a cheeky patient,' she said as she came away. 'Sometimes I'm not sure if he's teasing me or not.'

She answered the telephone. 'Talbot Ward, can I help you? No, I'm sorry, but he just went home, a short while ago. That's all right. Thank you for calling.' Then a porter came from theatres to call for a patient who had already gone, which caused a little confusion.

The sort of tension in this ward between two of the consultants and the nurses was not exceptional, but I never saw it in any of the other wards. Most of the doctors and consultants I spoke to in the course of the time I spent at the hospital were at great pains to talk a lot about the value of good and intelligent nurses, and the absolute importance of being on very good terms with them. On the whole the doctors boasted about how well they got on with the nursing staff, and how much attention they paid to their views but the nurses rarely mentioned it. At least most of the doctors were aware that the nurses mattered, even if they hadn't in fact got the relationship quite as right as they liked to imagine. Few of them really got beyond the stage of being sensitive to the feelings of those they still regarded as the lower orders.

The great barrier between doctors and nurses is still there, even though some nurses these days have university degrees. Until there is some integration of the two roles, with nurses able to ascend a scale towards becoming a doctor, with various grades of para-medical expertise in between, the barrier is likely to remain. At the moment, as with a great many other women's jobs, a nurse can only be promoted to an administrative position in charge of other nurses. This, it is often pointed out, is a disaster for the nursing profession, since it means that as soon as anyone gains real knowledge and experience in nursing, they are hurried away to a desk job, for which they may not be qualified at all. The better the nurse, the faster she will be promoted out of nursing, though many ward Sisters do long to teach. It is a waste of talent and skill. Most nurses are not at all happy with the way the system operates, but it is hard for anyone to turn down promotion when it comes.

At four o'clock, very tired, Anne came off duty. She wrapped her purple cloak around her. It was cold outside and we walked towards the back gate of the hospital. 'I do enjoy nursing, and I wouldn't want to do anything else – most of the time. But perhaps I've made it sound too easy? Have I painted you too rosy a picture? There are times, I'm sure any nurse will tell you, when you think you just can't keep going, you want to give it all up. I get terribly tired, and then I get fed up. A lot of things aren't the way you'd like them to be – but all the same, most of the time I think it's a great job.'

She pulled the cloak tighter round her shoulders and went off towards the nurses' home. I watched her go, and wondered what, in the last few days, she thought I'd seen that made her job seem too easy? Where was the rosy picture?

5

Casualty

The Emergency and Accident Department is a curious limbo land. It is more like a GP's practice than a part of the hospital. The patients look different. They are wearing their outside clothes, and in many ways don't appear to conform to the rules of patientdom. They are like unruly day pupils at a boarding school who have escaped the authority of the matrons.

I had imagined that this would have been one of the focal points of the life of the hospital – a place of drama, of lives being saved at the last minute, a place for quick and brilliant diagnoses in an hour of crisis. But most of the cases who amble quietly into the department are not at all like that.

I chose a Friday night to spend there. I was expecting at least one nearly-dead accident victim to be brought in for resuscitation but there were none that night. It was a quiet night, and at the end of it I was glad not to have had to witness anything too horrific. Many nurses in the hospital had said that they could stand to watch any kind of operation, but dealing with some of the worst cases that came in off the street was something else. I'd had enough graphic descriptions of crushed heads, severed limbs and gouged eyes to be grateful that this did not turn out to be one of the, on average, two nights a week when a serious emergency case came in.

I sat for a while with the receptionist at her desk at the entrance to the department. Lined up in front of her were rows of chairs, some of them occupied. An odd collection of people were sitting there, some waiting for treatment, most waiting for friends or relatives being treated. Further down the long room was a small partitioned office, where nurses and one or two doctors were sitting. Beyond that were rows of curtained cubicles with couches. Most of these were now empty, as it was still early, but some of them had the curtains drawn across.

There was a register on the desk – a big handwritten record of each person who came to the emergency department, a brief description of their complaint, and a note of whether they had been admitted to the hospital or discharged.

I looked through the last page to see who was being treated in the cubicles. There was an Indian Sikh with a badly lacerated middle finger, cut on a dress cutter. The hospital is in the centre of the East End rag trade. There was a girl who said she had fallen downstairs, and had a swollen nose. Her boy-friend was waiting for her in one of the chairs, looking morose and fidgety. There was a woman who had stuck a sewing machine needle in her arm two days before, and now suddenly her arm had swollen up. There was a middle-aged man, a regular customer, the receptionist said, who had slashed his wrist yet again, though not very badly.

The receptionist surveyed the scene in front of us, and in a quiet voice explained who all the waiting people were. At the back of the chairs, in a corner was a derelict old man, asleep, and nodded so far over in his chair that his head nearly touched the floor. I wondered how long it would be before he toppled forwards. 'He's a wino, a meths drinker,' she said in half a whisper. 'He's been sitting there for two hours now.' I asked what he was waiting for. 'Well, he's one of those old tramps from Victoria House [a local Salvation Army hostel]. He came in here and asked to see a doctor because he wanted some drugs.'

'What kind?' I asked.

'Oh, any kind. He said his head hurt, then his stomach. He just wanted anything he could get. The doctor sent him away, but he wouldn't go.'

'Do you just let them sit there?' I asked.

'If they don't cause any trouble, we turn a blind eye. It often causes more trouble to ask them to leave. We thought if we let him sit he'd get bored in the end and go away. He thinks if he sits there long enough the doctors will give in. It's a kind of battle of wills.'

'Does he want to be admitted for the night?' I asked.

'Yes. Most of them know that's not on, but they do try. Of course the doctors have to be very careful, because often they really are ill.'

A trolley was wheeled past from one of the cubicles out to the main part of the hospital. On it was a very young woman, half propped up on pillows crying so that her make-up had smudged down her cheeks. Just behind her came her young husband trailing two small children who were both howling too.

'What's the matter with her?' I asked. She looked in the book. It said, 'Incomplete abortion.' Abortion in medical terminology simply means a miscarriage of any kind, not neccessarily intentionally induced. She was wheeled away to a gynaecological ward.

Three young men came in through the doors, laughing together. A fat young boy of about sixteen came up to the desk, holding his hand in front of his mouth. 'Can I help you?' asked the receptionist.

'I've smashed my teeth,' he said. He took away his hand and showed that his mouth was bloody and his three front teeth bent right inwards. He didn't appear to be in pain, or to be very upset. 'We were doing judo in the club and I was thrown on my face,' he said. 'They sent me up here.' He gave his name and address and she told him to wait.

Just as these boys had sat down, another group of giggly young people came in. There were three girls and two boys from a local commune. The girls were wearing long Indian print dresses and shawls, the boys had their hair in plaits down their backs. They all talked at once 'We've been clearing out this old butcher's shop,' one said. 'We were cleaning up an old fridge when this stuff started leaking out of the bottom.'

Another said, 'We felt really queer, sort of faint.'

'I started seeing things, very odd things,' said a third. 'I'd read somewhere about gas fridges having dangerous chemicals in them and I got us all out of there. I nearly fainted, and I still feel sick.' The receptionist hesitated before writing in the book, 'Poisoning from fridge', and then took all their names and addresses.

Further down the room, in one of the cubicles an old drunk was being lifted out of a wheelchair back onto a couch. He had just been sent for an X-ray. The young woman doctor on duty was worried about his chest and suspected TB. He was shouting at the top of his voice, 'I want to go home!'

A nurse was with him; she smiled and said, 'But you can't even walk!' The doctor went into the cubicle to talk to him, to tell him she was worried about his chest, but he was too drunk to listen. 'He's a regular. I know this gentleman,' the nurse said.

'Doctor, I want to go home,' said the man again.

'Where do you live?' the doctor asked.

'Never you mind. I'll call my son. He'll come and get me.' The doctor asked where his son lived.

'Weston-Super-Mare,' said the man, and they left him there, hoping he would quieten down and sleep until the X-ray results came back. He was another Victoria House inmate.

There is a professor who is responsible for the two Emergency and Accident Departments. Fourteen other doctors work in the department and at Mile End for six months at a time. The hours are shorter and more regular, so these posts usually go to people studying for exams. It is considered a good starting job for a young doctor, perhaps because it is more like general practice than any other job in the hospital as it cuts across all specialties. For any serious case that comes into the department at night, the relevant specialist can be called out of bed.

A mountainously fat old woman was being taken into one of the cubicles and laid upon the couch by a pair of strong ambulance drivers. The woman's middle-aged daughter was with her, carrying a small attaché case. The senior doctor looked out of his office and saw her. He caught the arm of the young doctor who was about to go to her and said, 'I know her. You'll find she has massive notes. She was in Devonshire Ward for a long time, a few months back.' He clicked his fingers and shut his eyes, trying to remember her name; 'Ah, it's Mrs Besom!' he said. The young doctor went in to talk to her. She groaned loudly, and swore at him when he gently lifted one of her legs. A while later he came out, and said he was confused by her symptoms. She was clearly suffering very acute abdominal pain. He said, 'Query intestinal blockage?'

The SHO said he'd look at her. 'She has a multiple pathology, everything wrong with her you care to imagine. He went into her cubicle and smiled at her, 'Hello, old friend!' he said.

'Piss off!' she hissed back at him.

'But you remember me, don't you, Mrs Besom, from Devonshire Ward?'

'Yes, course I do. Get off out of it!' The daughter hurried up to apologize for her mother's behaviour. The SHO smiled at her, told her not to worry, and proceeded to examine her mother.

An ambulanceman with a clipboard came up to the Staff Nurse in the office. 'What have you brought us, Bill?' she asked. The nurses here knew almost all the ambulancemen, and many of the local police too.

'Just this one. He was down in the gutter, said he hurt his elbow.'

'Drunk?' asked the nurse.

'You bet,' said the driver. 'I'm afraid we had to be a bit rough with him to get him in. He came up fighting.' They wheeled him into a cubicle and put him onto a bed. 'Want us to hang around, see he doesn't start any funny business again?' one ambulanceman asked.

'No, it's all right. We'll manage,' said the nurse and smiled as the two men went off. She went into the cubicle, pulling the curtains shut behind her, and started to undress the man. When it came to taking off his shoes and socks, the smell was apalling. His socks looked as if they hadn't been taken off for a very long time – they were stiff with accumulated sweat and grime. His shirt too was filthy, and he had been sick down the front of it, and on his jacket. But the young nurse didn't seem to mind. 'Oh, good heavens, you get used to it!' she said and laughed at my disgust. The man mumbled and sometimes yelled abuse at her when she touched the arm that hurt, but she was tolerant.

'Don't you get sick of all these drunks?' I asked, surprised by the remarkable tolerance of all the nurses in the department.

'Well, it's not their fault, is it? Either we get the young men, not used to the drink, out on a once-only binge, and you can't be too hard on them for that. They'll get their punishment when they come round. Or you get the addicts, and you have to be sorry for them.' I agreed. I could understand that theoretically she was right, but if it was me clearing up the vomit I shouldn't have been so philosophical about it. A doctor came to see him, and after examining him, as best he could, or dared, he ordered him to be taken for an X-ray of his arm. When the porters came he swore at them and threatened his good fist, but they bundled him into the chair and wheeled him off.

A porter arrived with a packet of ham sandwiches ordered by one of the doctors. Some more ambulancemen brought in a fattish man in his late thirties with a very badly cut lip. The driver told the nurse the name of the factory they had collected him from. A large industrial spring had leapt up and smashed his face. The bottom part of his lip looked as if it had turned inside out, and bled a lot. He leant on one arm on the couch in his cubicle, and smiled sheepishly at the nurse, unable to speak more than a painful word or two.

There was a loud crash in a cubicle further down the room. The drunk who had had his chest X-ray for TB had fallen onto the ground. A nurse hurried in to see if he was all right. He had taken off all his clothes, and was lying totally naked, sprawled across the floor. He was extraordinarily thin. His hip bones protruded sharply from his thin bright white skin and his ribs looked jagged. His toe-nails were twisted and black, and at his wrist and his neck was a dramatic change of colour. His face and hands were reddish brown from living so much of his life out on the streets, and the rest of his body was so white it was almost blue. The nurse tried to get him up. 'Would you like to sit up?' she said.

The man groaned and then said, 'No! I'll stay here!' He had knocked over his urine bottle and there was a large puddle on the floor.

'Well, you're going to get up, my man,' said the nurse with firmness, heaving him from under his arms. He was not heavy to lift, a bundle of bones. He shouted at her again so in the end she said, 'Well, I'll have to leave you there then,' and she threw a blanket over him and fetched a mop to clean the floor.

The other drunk with the bad arm was trundled in by a porter. 'He hit the radiographer, and she couldn't do him,' the porter told a nurse, who just sighed, and told him to put the man in a cubicle and leave him in his chair for the moment since he seemed to be sleeping.

A tall anxious-looking young man came into the department in a white coat. He hesitated outside the nurses' office. 'Are you the oral surgeon we sent for?' asked the Staff Nurse. He said he was. He looked at his notes and said he'd come to see a Mr Fulton. She showed him to the cubicle containing the man with the lacerated lower lip. 'We don't really know the dentists very well,' she explained to me. 'And he's a new one.'

The young boy who had smashed his teeth at judo was brought back from X-ray. The girl radiographer said to the oral surgeon, who was also to treat this patient, 'His tooth fell out. It was while I was doing the X-ray.'

'Where is it then?' asked the stiff young oral surgeon.

'I threw it away,' said the radiographer. The surgeon looked vexed.

'I wanted to *see* it,' he said. The radiographer looked a little sour and said she'd go and see if she could retrieve it. The oral surgeon went back to his examination of the man with the cut lip.

Then came a short girl with cropped black hair, wearing a stripey blue and white shirt, the back and shoulders of which were splattered with blood. There was a lot of blood all over her, but she didn't look distressed. Her-boy friend, a West Indian, was with her, looking sheepish. The nurse explained to the doctor, after she had shown the girl to a cubicle that the boy had broken a glass over his girl-friend's head in a fight in a pub. He was sorry now, and she didn't seem to be cross with him. The doctor came to examine the cut. 'It's not very big,' he said, and he pulled back the dyed roots of her hair, now solidly matted with blood. 'But it's quite deep.' He led her down to the dentist's chair at the far end of the room, where he sat her down and shone the bright arc lamp on her head. He called for the suture trolley and started to stitch her up. She chatted to him as he did it, and her boy-friend, after a while, came and sat beside her, and soon they were all talking and sometimes laughing together. One of the things I found most admirable, and most remarkable about the doctors and nurses working in this department was their complete lack of any moral judgement on the patients they were treating and their friends. They regarded the nature of the accident as not being in any way their business. It didn't seem to require any self-control in them not to lecture, reprimand or demand explanations. They ministered to their patients without appearing to make any distinction at all.

An amublanceman, accompanied by a policeman, brought in another drunk. This time it was a young boy of fifteen, quite unconscious. The policeman said he'd been called in by people at the party this boy had been at. The boy had, as a dare, drunk eighteen vodkas in a row, was sick five times and then passed straight out. He'd been brought to the hospital as his friends had been worried. They thought he had vomited a lot of blood. He was covered in vomit, all over his fashionable green baggy trousers and skintight jersey. The policeman gave the boy's name, Barry Stephens, and his address and phone number. The nurses offered the policeman and the ambulanceman a cup of coffee in the rest room at the far end of the room, beyond the dentist's chair. A nurse went to undress Barry. She stripped off his outer clothes and put them in a polythene bag, which she sealed. She called his name, slapped his cheeks, and he groaned and his eyes flickered. 'Wake up Barry! Wake up! You're in hospital! You've had a bit too much to drink! Come on, boy, open your eyes.' He retched and she fetched him a small bowl. He clung to the edge of the bed, looking very young and vulnerable. 'Poor lad!' she said. A doctor examined him, but they all agreed there was no cause for concern. It later emerged that he had been drinking bloody marys and had vomited not blood, but tomato juice.

A man called Michael who had tried to kill himself suddenly awoke in the next-door cubicle and he began to cry and rock himself about on his bed. A young doctor went in and sat by him. The man had blood stains all down the cuff of his left arm. Some matted blood clung to his wrist where he had cut it but the cut was superficial and would not even need stitches. There were countless old scars on his wrists, many more on the left than the right, showing he was right handed. 'Hello, Michael,' said the doctor. 'I'm sorry to see you here again,' he said.

The man began to cry again. 'I'm an ex-soldier,' he was saying between sobs. 'I've served all over the world, a good soldier. Then I served in Ireland too. It's more than I could stand, I'm telling you. What was I to do? My own countrymen killing each other, for nothing, nothing!' His words were barely audible between sobs. He rambled on indistinctly.

The Staff Nurse put her head round the door and called to the doctor to come out for a moment. 'You were away last week,' she said in a loud whisper. 'You missed what happened with him. He slashed his wrist, right here in the department. We left him alone for just a minute or two, and he had a razor blade in his pocket. It was quite a drama, I can tell you.'

There was another crash from another cubicle. The man with the bad arm had toppled out of his wheelchair onto the floor. A nurse bustled in to see if he was all right. 'You all right?' she asked him.

'No, I'm not fucking all right,' he said, just raising his head a few inches off the floor to give her a nasty look. 'I don't feel very well just now. Will you GO AWAY!' So she went, and left him there.

A drunken jolly group of people had come into the department roaring with laughter, and tottering against one another. There was a tousled young girl, with her mother, and her older boy-friend who was carrying a tiny puppy on one arm, and the girl's father who was very drunk indeed. 'Nurse!' called the girl's boy-friend. 'Where are you, nurse?' They tottered down the room. 'We're here, wa-hey!' he whooped and they all collapsed in giggles on the front row of chairs. They had used up their last bit of sobriety and self-control in the massive effort of getting themselves to the hospital. The puppy whimpered and clung to the man's arm. The reception-ist had gone home, as it was long past ten-thirty now, so a nurse came to take their details. It took some minutes to sort out which was the patient. It turned out that the young girl had cut her wrist on a broken milk bottle after having a row with her boy-friend. They'd all forgotten what the row was about.

'I did it a few hours ago,' she said vaguely. The nurse looked at her wrist.

'You're very lucky it's not cut an artery, or you'd be dead by now, taking so long to get here.' They laughed some more, as the girl was led to a cubicle to have stitches put in the cut.

Then came an anxious young woman with her mother. She was four months pregnant, had started to bleed a little that day and was afraid she would have a miscarriage. One of the nurses said to another nurse that the girl should have gone to her own doctor in the daytime, but the other said sym-pathetically, 'You tend to worry more at night.'

One of the surprising things was the number of people who dared to walk into a big hospital with the most trivial com-plaints, because they couldn't be bothered to register with a doctor. In the course of the evening several people had come in with tooth-ache. There used to be a dentist on duty all the time, and people still expected there to be one in the department. But the service was abused, and people who couldn't be bothered to make an appointment and go to their own dentist would wait till the evening and go to the department for small cavities. 'This hospital has always been treated like that. It's partly because in the East End the GP service is erratic. Almost all the GPs live a long way out of the district. It has become a sort of tradition. This is their hospital, they feel, and they think they have the right to come in for anything any time,' one of the doctors explained. That night three people came in to see if they could get repeat prescriptions from the hospital pharmacy, because they'd forgotten to get them during the day from a chemist. They were told the address of a far-away all-night chemist and each left after much grumbling. Two people came in with mild 'flu, and several people with accidents that had happened some time ago.

A snazzily dressed young man came next, looking extremely anxious. A nurse led him to a cubicle to take his particulars. He had been waiting for some time, but everyone had assumed he was waiting for one of the patients, since he just sat there, and didn't push himself at all. The nurse came out and reported to a doctor. 'He's complaining of chest pains, and shaking all over. He thinks he's got VD. He didn't say it very nicely, but that's what he means.' The doctor went in to examine him. The nurse said to another, 'He looks familiar to me. Does he to you? Has he been here before?' She peeked through the curtains at him, and agreed he did look familiar.

One of the ambulancemen came back from having a cup of tea. He had picked Michael the suicide man up earlier in the evening and he looked in on him to see how he was. 'Remember me?' he said. 'How are you feeling now?'

Michael, tried to sit up and look at him. 'You're a good man, a good man,' he said blurrily to the driver.

The driver answered 'What do you want to go and do a thing like that for, eh? There's a lot to live for, you know.'

Michael just shook his head and mumbled, 'I like you, for you're a good man.' Then he said, with tears falling again, 'Stay with me, son, just for a while? My mind's in a terrible state, terrible.'

The ambulanceman sat beside him and took his hand. 'If you knew what I knew, you'd be doing it too,' Michael said delphicly.

'Not me, mate,' said the ambulanceman. 'Life's too good for me.'

'Ah, what do you know of life? You're a simple man, and you may thank the good Lord for that blessing!' Michael said with passion.

The ambulanceman tried to calm him by saying firmly, 'Do you ever stop and count your blessings, Michael. You've a lot going for you, if you only add it up. You're a good-looking chap, and you've got your health. Why throw it away?'

Michael groaned, sank back on the pillows and said, 'I hope you keep your innocence.'

The ambulanceman smiled and said he must be going. 'Keep your pecker up,' he said. Michael smiled back to him.

As the ambulanceman came out, a doctor who had been waiting outside the curtain and had heard the conversation asked him with some surprise in his voice, 'Did you know him before? Are you a friend of his?'

The ambulanceman shook his head. 'I don't know him from Adam, mate. And you know, the funny thing is, when we went to pick him up he was fighting, real hard, and we both got knocked about a bit, but he seems to have forgotten that now.' The doctor looked a little pained, the ambulanceman laughed and turned to go, but then he stopped, and called to someone near by. 'Here, I'd better give these to you, I suppose. Look what I just found in his pocket. Didn't you search him, even after what happened last time he was in?' The ambulanceman dropped a large pair of scissors into the embarrassed person's hand, and then a necktie, and walked out of the department whistling.

Barry, the young drunk boy, was being sat up in bed, and a nurse was talking to him again. 'You're all right to go home, then?' she said. He mumbled that he wanted to sleep. 'Well you can't sleep the night here. We'll ring your parents, and put you in a taxi. Have you the money for a taxi?' He said he had. She went away to call for a taxi, but one firm after another, enquiring nervously as to what sort of case they were to be taking, refused, or said they couldn't manage it. They were all wary of late-night rejects from the emergency department. She sighed and gave up for the moment. Barry had gone comfortably back to sleep. She then tried ringing the police, since they had brought him in, but they too refused to take him home.

A middle-aged Indian woman came in with her teenage daughter. She didn't speak a word of English and her daughter translated for her. Her husband had hit her hard a day or two ago. It had been painful since then, but was now suddenly agonizing. She had kept away from the hospital as long as she could, for fear of getting her husband into trouble. Finally her daughter had insisted on bringing her in. It turned out she had a bad fracture.

Horace, the young boy, had a temperature which seemed to be going up every half-hour. They kept him on his couch for observation. They couldn't get his notes at this time of night, (though if it had been a real emergency they would have) but one of the doctors remembered his having attended the skin clinic regularly. They all agreed there was something odd about him. Several nurses then remembered him having come into the department regularly with one complaint or another. The doctor was worried about his chest. Eventually he was admitted, though no one had a very satisfactory diagnosis. They agreed he was deeply neurotic. They didn't think he did have VD after all.

The psychiatrist who had been summoned out of bed from St Clement's hospital to see Michael at last arrived. He was a Persian doctor, and Michael appeared to take against him. After a brief conversation the psychiatrist decided to admit him, and he was taken away later, when he was sober enough to go into a ward without causing too much trouble.

'I feel more hotter and hotter!' Horace suddenly burst out,

in a panic, and a nurse went to calm him. He seemed to be getting hysterical, and they decided to try to get him to sleep there, and send him to the ward in the morning. 'It's not fair on the night staff in the wards, and we try not to send them noisy cases if we can help it,' a nurse said.

Someone came from the plaster room to say that they couldn't get the bangles off the Indian woman's arm to plaster it. No one had a metal cutter, so they considered calling the fire brigade to see if they could help. The police and fire brigade seemed to enjoy the chance of a visit to the hospital late at night. They got bored sitting around, and were glad of a coffee and a laugh with the nurses.

A man came in with three strong-looking friends. He was still shaking with anger. He had a thick beard, but even under that you could see there was something odd about his face. He had broken his jaw, or at least someone else had broken it for him. 'Bumped into a door,' he said. He was taken to sit in the dentist's chair, and the oral surgeon was summoned from bed for the second time that night. I got the feeling that it gave the night doctors and nurses a kind of wicked pleasure to have to call sleeping specialists from their beds in the early hours of the morning, to see how the other half lived.

The man was muttering with his friends. He told one of the nurses that they'd better hurry up and fix him up as he'd got some, 'Very, very important business to see to tonight, and it can't wait till morning.' He said it between clenched teeth since he couldn't move his jaw, and he had a thunderous, murderous look in his eye.

His friends nodded their heads and one said, 'That's right. Very important business with a certain party, or parties.' The nurses laughed at them and told them not to talk such silly nonsense, 'boys' talk' one of them said, and got a dirty look from the three. One of the nurses couldn't help laughing when they were out of earshot.

'I shouldn't like to be the one to tell him he's probably got to stay in here a month, and that he's going to have to have his jaws wired together in the operating theatre tomorrow.' When he was told, his friends slunk off, hands in jacket pockets and one of them muttered to the nurses that they had better go off and do their 'very important business' without their friend, since 'it definitely won't wait till morning'.

I asked a nurse if they would warn the police of the probable battle. 'Oh no,' said a nurse very sensibly. 'Those overgrown teddy boys are far too drunk to hurt a flea. Anyway, they've been here two hours now and I doubt there's a man with a sore fist waiting around in the same place for a sore jaw too!'

The radiographer came in a while later to grumble about the nastiness of the patients they'd sent her that night. 'Is getting hit part of the job, do you think?' she asked, but she laughed good-naturedly. The two drunks were still fast asleep on the floor of their cubicles. She pointed at the one with the bad arm who she had failed to X-ray. 'He was the worst, but the jaw case had a nasty lip. I'd have stitched his mouth up if I'd have been you!' The drunk with the bad arm roused himself, peed into his bottle and then dropped it with a crash.

'Now look what you've done!' said one of the nurses, coming in with a mop, and a bucket.

'I didn't piss the floor,' he said slowly.

'What's all this then?' she asked as she cleaned up around him.

'I didn't piss the floor,' he said again. She touched his bare toes with the mop and he swore. 'I DIDN'T PISS THE FLOOR!' he bellowed, and all the nurses were laughing.

6

Consultant

Mr West was one of the top consultants at The London Hospital. He was an orthopaedic surgeon of international repute, famous for his treatment of hips, knees and ankles. He was one of the hospital's stars, one of the high-flyers that have always given British teaching hospitals their great prestige all over the world. Many foreign doctors came to study under him and to observe his work.

He was not a 'typical' consultant in the hospital's terms, as so much of his time was taken up with his research. Also he had a thriving private practice, which most of the consultants at the hospital do not. His contract with the National Health was that he should carry out seven of a notional maximum of eleven sessions clinically for the Service. His week divided up as one and a half days in his laboratory doing research, half a day in his consulting rooms in Harley Street and visiting his patients in the London Clinic, and three days at The London, where he had an out-patient clinic, conducted operations and carried out ward rounds for the National Health. He also fitted into those three days a private clinic and some private operations in Fielden House, the private wing at The London.

On top of all this he found time for active membership of the Medical Research Council, the body which decides how to allocate government research funds, assessing different projects and their ultimate usefulness to medicine. He also carried out clinical teaching sessions with the medical students at The London, and he frequently gave lectures all over the country.

He often travelled abroad to lecture and to attend medical conferences. Work consumed most of his life. His wife spent much of her time running the administrative side of his private practice.

'Mr West' is not his real name. After I had written this chapter he alone of all the doctors in the book decided he would prefer, after all, to remove his name. Mr West's main reason for wishing to to be anonymous is that doctors are forbidden to advertise in any way. Since I have described his Harley Street private practice, and the hospital where he is to be found most of the time, he feels this amounts to advertising, and that he should therefore have his name removed.

One Monday morning I found him in his laboratory. It had Bio-Mechanics written on the door. Descending the noisy metal stairs I could survey the room below, light and airy — with presses and machines, sinks and equipment all round the room, and amongst all this several technicians and researchers were working. At the foot of the stairs was a large refrigerator·

'Hope you've got a strong stomach, not too squeamish?' Mr West had enquired with a casual bluffness on the telephone. I said I hoped so too.

Mr West had taken off his jacket and had rolled the sleeves of his shirt to the elbow. He was standing at a bench near a sink. His technician, Bill, was standing beside him.

'Let's get started,' he said to Bill, after introductions. He went over to the sink in which was standing a large polythene bag, partly in soak, in which were a collection of frozen knees. They had been cut off a good six inches each side of the joint, no blood but yellow fatty tissue protruding.

Picking out a good knee from the bag, Mr West clamped it firmly into position to operate on. He was experimenting with a new shape for his patent prosthesis, a plastic covering that fits onto the shin bone, and another metal piece that fits onto the thigh bone. It is used for people with damaged and arthritic knee joints, where the cartilage has worn away and the bones grind painfully against each other.

Bill said something off-hand about the shortage of good cadavers in the fridge, but I think they were only bits of bodies, just hips, knees and ankles.

With the knee in the right place, West cut away the skin and fat and began to saw the top off the shin bone, ready to receive the plastic piece. The electric saw made a low scream. He drilled two holes in the side of the bone and the marrow oozed out. This was a different shaped prosthesis from the one currently in use. It had two plastic prongs that were pushed down into the bone, in the hope that when the bone grew again it would grow round and into the plastic, keeping it more strongly in position.

A young American doctor had been sent to study West's methods, and was working for six months in the laboratory. He came over to watch. 'We in the States were embarrassed by discovering that our version of this doesn't work properly so I was sent over to study here,' he explained.

West carefully fitted the prosthesis over the hole he had cut. 'A dead fit!' he exclaimed. 'Oh I'm happy about that one, very chuffed!' He then cemented it into place with a nasty-smelling glue.

The young American had gone back to a huge press in the middle of the room. He was testing an ankle joint he had just fitted. The large bone, with the joint in the middle was sticking out of the middle of the press. By pulling on a lever he could exert pressure, measured on a dial and could gauge the strength of the joint and its breaking point. He warned us to stand back lest the joint break up and send jagged pieces of bone shooting across the room.

'The art of surgery,' Mr West said, without looking up while he wrenched at some cartilage in the knee, 'is getting at the piece of the body you want, getting it into a good position for drilling or sawing without at the same time doing terrible harm to anything else. It's no good having your patients waking up covered in bruises or sometimes worse.'

He pulled off his rubber gloves and began to wash his hands thoroughly. 'Well Bill, I'm pleased,' he said over his shoulder. 'I'll leave it to you for the torsion tests.'

We went upstairs to his office. There he explained that the first knee joint using metal and polythene had been fitted some five years before, almost simultaneously invented by himself and a Canadian in the UK. Since then he had worked steadily on improving it.

He set to work on his mail. Someone in Germany wanted to translate and print his work *Adult Articular Cartilage*. A Japanese surgeon had written to ask permission to use a smaller version of his patented knee on elderly Japanese, as his knees were too big for Japanese patients.

A German manufacturer wanted to make his hips and knees in ceramic. There was a letter about his forthcoming paper to be read to the US Academy of Orthopedic Surgery, which invites one foreigner a year to speak, and then confers on him an Honorary Fellowship. The University of Leeds was offering him a paltry £15 plus expenses to give a lecture. He had a waiting list of at least a year for out-of-town lectures, but he accepted the Leeds invitation.

He suddenly stopped dictating and leant back in his chair, tipping it and stretching his legs. (I couldn't help looking at his knees, thin and pointy. Knees had taken on a new dimension.)

'This laboratory and our work at The London now have an international reputation. We're amongst the top two or three. But can we maintain it? That's the question. The Health Service is about to pack up, and if it does, the clinical base for all this will disappear. If there is no research there will be a total collapse of morale. No, I wouldn't leave the country. There are a few of us who wouldn't. I like living in England, but I dread to think what medicine will be like.' He paused, tapping his pen on the desk top.

'A hospital is like a warship in the face of battle. If the crew is mutinous, however good the guns, it's no use. It will almost become unsafe to bring patients into hospital if we can't depend on the staff, if there may be a strike at any time,' he said.

He was referring to an overtime dispute which was causing trouble at the time. The hospital's engineers had started an overtime ban. The Administration had sent out directives to all consultants to admit only emergency cases. The laundry had ceased to function effectively and there was a severe linen shortage. The orthopaedic department suffered particularly since many of their admissions couldn't easily be categorized as emergencies. There was a lot of wheeling and dealing going between the consultants. I was with Dr Goodwin of the nephrology department one day during the dispute. He was pacing the wards, whispering to the Sisters. In one of his wards he found that a prudent Sister had stockpiled a vast amount of linen, plenty to keep his non-emergency admissions flowing. The Sister was anxious that he shouldn't tell the Administration that she had all this extra linen, as she wanted to keep it for her ward. 'Do you think we could? Could we just admit a few, do you think?' he asked her conspiratorially. He went down to the Administrators in the end, and being careful not to disclose the ward in question said, 'If I found the linen could I keep admitting my patients?' There was a fairly indignant no from Administration, who were hard put to find enough linen for their emergencies. Dr Goodwin huffed off, in a bad temper, and no doubt the Administrators ordered a quick search of some of the ward linen stocks.

I include this small anecdote as it shows how consultants operate in complete isolation from the rest of the hospital. The hospital is not one organization, but a collection of empires in angry competition with each other for beds, money, machines and other resources. This is not an idle metaphor, but the truth. There is no one higher than the consultants, no higher authority. The Administrators are the mere servants of the kings. They co-ordinate, and try to keep the building and the non-medical staff functioning. They cannot interfere in any way with how consultants run their kingdoms. Nor can they make serious priority judgements between departments. The

District Management Team decides who should get large sums of money under much pressure from consultants lobbying. But the consultant in his own department is autonomous. Only he decides how many patients are seen in out-patient clinics. Since re-organization and the passing of the old authoritarian House Governor, a new brand of dynamic young Administrators fresh out of hospital administration courses has taken over, but they are without power, respect, or seniority. They are only housekeepers, not house governors, and they have a hard time.

The consultants are left to fight it out amongst themselves in a series of complicated and unsatisfactory committees. Each of them strives to increase the size of their domain. Few, it seems, have any consideration for the general good of all patients, only, putting it at its best, caring for the rights of their own patients.

There is a belief amongst doctors, unassailable and inviolable, that nothing, no authority in the world must come between them and their patients. They and only they must have complete freedom to prescribe the right treatment. It is on this basis that the consultants can build around them such powerful empires. There is no one above or below them to challenge their authority.

It was over lunch that day that Mr West discussed this point. 'I regard the Health Service as nothing more than a mechanism for paying for the medical care of the patients, a sort of insurance, and nothing more. We consultants have no loyalties whatever to the Health Service, nor should we. All our loyalties are to our patients and the hospital. Things are getting quite out of hand now though.'

I asked about the accountability of consultants. 'Oh you can't get rid of a consultant, not once he's been appointed. There is no procedure for removing him, unless of course he starts killing off a noticeably large number of people. But it's difficult even then. There was once a surgeon who was absolutely senile, poor man. It was a devil of a job getting him to go. A lot of consultants are very lazy and sloppy. But there is no one anywhere who is in a position to examine the quality of his work, the number of patients he bothers to treat, the amount of teaching he bothers to do, or how up to date he is with new developments in his field.'

Mr West, however, saw no easy way in which consultants could, or perhaps should be made accountable. His fear of state intervention in medicine was far greater than his disapproval of the erratic behaviour and internecine disputes between warring consultants.

Mr West's ward round began at 9.30 in the morning, the group collecting together at the doorway of Cotton Ward. He had already started the morning with a teaching session of the medical students attached to his 'firm' at the time. He also had with him two foreign doctors who were spending some time with him to learn his special techniques before returning to their own countries. One was Australian, one American.

The group stood around for a time at the head of the ward discussing some new research that Mr West was currently engaged in — much talk of grinding down on minimal shifts, quadriceps, medial pivotal shifts, patellas and rotation of the knee. 'Yes, I'm turned on by that idea, I really am,' Mr West was saying. 'But don't for heaven's sake regard it as an absolute dictum, a tablet of stone, yet.'

I puzzled often over why so many of the doctors were so good looking. In almost all the departments where I went the doctors, especially the grander ones were handsome. I evolved a theory that their own bodily perfections had led them into medicine and the study of how bodies work. I doubt there's any truth in it. I often heard the nurses grumble about the narcissism and excessive self-confidence of the doctors. When I asked one doctor once he said he thought it was all built into the selection process. Doctors selecting prospective medical students had a predilection for the best and most beautiful of the species.

The discussion of the new knee was now over, and, led by

Mr West, the group now moved off to the beginning of the ward round.

Two-thirds of Mr West's patients came under what he termed 'elective surgery' and one-third were emergencies. The emergencies were mainly old people with hip fractures. The others are people with damaged or arthritic hips, knees, feet or other joints. 'Elective' makes it sound as if it is mainly cosmetic, but most of the patients were in great pain, some severely crippled before they were operated on. What makes it 'elective' is that it is not *absolutely* essential; the patients will not die without it.

Cotton Ward was a women's surgical ward, light and bright, an exact replica of most of the other wards in the hospital – T-shaped in layout. In the first bed was a lady in her mid sixties. As they approached, Mr West smiled broadly at her and he said, 'Good morning, my dear, how are you?' The woman pulled herself up, smiled warmly and said she wasn't too good. 'How's the walking?'

'Oh, terrible,' she answered.

The physiotherapist, who was hovering in the background, came forward and said, 'Well, she's had a little toddle today.'

Mr West asked the woman to get out of bed. Helped by a nurse, and holding with one hand on to the chain dangling above her, she swung her legs over the side of the bed, and slowly got to her feet. They looked odd, with thick pads on the soles, so her toes were raised two or three inches off the ground. She had bad arthritis in her feet, which had distorted her bones, making them grow downwards. She had just been operated on to have some of the bone removed.

'Try and push your toes downwards,' he said, as she tottered for a moment, with her bare feet on the lino, one arm clutching the nurse. 'Does it hurt you now?' he asked.

'OOOH yes! Like cramp,' she answered.

'Well of course, it will for a while. You've got cut bones and they do hurt. But you must try and walk through that. The pain is only temporary. Now go on, quick march!' She had a stick now and was walking slowly unassisted, with a nurse at her elbow to catch her should she fall. 'Smashing!' he said. 'But look up. Don't look at your feet. I know when you look up it feels as if you'll fall, but you won't. Now, I want you to pick up your left foot, as high as you can,' he said.

She lifted it and then said, 'Oooh!' again.

'And the right,' he persisted and she said, 'That gives me cramp, in both of them.' Mr West said she was much better though, and doing well. 'I shan't see you again in here,' he said to her. 'I shan't be here next week, as I've got to go to Madrid and do some amazing things to Spaniards, and by the time I get back you'll have gone home, so I'll say good-bye, and see you in out-patients.' She said good-bye, rather painfully as she was manoeuvring herself back into bed.

In the next bed was a youngish woman with one leg in plaster, except for a square window-hole at the knee. Mr West exchanged a friendly word or two with her. A nurse approached him and said there was a call for him, from the Iranian Embassy. 'Tell them I'm tied up and I'll call them later,' he said. He turned back to the woman and noticed she was wearing a pair of pants. 'Good heavens!' he said and laughed. 'However did you get them on? I've never known anyone be able to do that before!' He then said he would like to cut away a larger piece of the plaster and a young nurse went off to get some scissors. He tried to cut it off, but the plaster was too thick. The nurse went to fetch some special shears, and Mr West left a young doctor hacking away at the leg, saying he would be back when they'd got the plaster off.

In the next bed was a classic case of the kind he had to deal with every week. A very old frail lady was lying quite still. She was rather deaf, and according to one of the young doctors, also vague and confused. Mr West spoke a word or two to her, but relied for communication with her on holding her hand for a minute or two and smiling reassuringly to her while they discussed her case. Her long grey hair was arrayed on the pillow. She had fallen and broken her hip.

'It's as thin as eggshell, very difficult to deal with, but we pinned it,' said the young Australian doctor, who had kindly taken it on himself to explain the cases to me as we progressed round the ward.

'Is she walking?' Mr West asked. The nurse said she wasn't. 'Well, you've just got to get her going, any way you can. It is most important that we get her out of bed.'

The young Australian said the trouble was, that in cases like this it was very difficult to get the patient walking, but absolutely essential. By one fall on a hip an old person, independent and managing alone could be transformed into an institutionalized cripple. 'We call this "the inevitable fracture",' he whispered. 'The trouble is, they lie around in hospital beds for weeks and months. It would be cheaper to transport them to the Hilton, it really would, I'm not joking.'

Mr West went back to the woman with her leg in plaster. The shears too had made no impression, so he called for an electric drill. As he raised it, turned it on, and the big rotary blade approached her leg, the woman blanched, understandably, and screwed up her eyes. 'Don't worry. It isn't going to touch your leg. I'd demonstrate on my own knee, if it was in plaster.' He then carried out the examination and pronounced himself pleased with the results.

The next woman had been a patient of Mr West's for many years. She must have sampled almost every aspect of his surgical skills. She suffered badly from rheumatoid arthritis. She was in her early forties, a pretty, delicate woman, with dark hair elegantly and finely streaked with white. She had a pale and anxious face. After a friendly greeting, Mr West looked at her foot. The toes were twisted, and there were scars where she had been operated on. He pressed her big toe, and watched it blanch, then redden when he took his finger away. 'Now there's something to make you happy!' he said to the two doctors, and they nodded. Blanching was a very good sign. She had had a polythene ball-bearing put into her big-toe joint to make walking easier. By her feet were two rubber gloves tied at the ends and filled with water. They looked oddly sinister, but were good for resting under heels in danger of developing pressure sores.

Mr West was examining her stitches. He squeezed together the two sides of the wound, and it oozed a little. He squeezed again, and mopped it. Arthritics tend to have problems with the healing of their wounds after operations. 'I think we're going to have to re-suture and neaten the edges of that,' he said. He addressed the woman, 'That will be the quickest way to get it to heal, if we can re-stitch it. You had a knee done last year, didn't you, and we had a little trouble with that healing too.'

She cleared her throat and asked, 'Excuse me, but this stitching, will I have to go down to the theatre again?' (The patients, significantly, always referred to the operating theatres as 'down'.)

'Yes, you will,' he answered. 'It'll just be a brief operation.'

'Will I be opened up again?' she asked.

'No, I don't think so,' he said. She had already had both hips, both knees and both hands operated on. Her hands were still distorted, like her feet. The young Australian said she had been bowed right over on one side before her hips had been done. He said no one knew what rheumatoid arthritis was, or what caused it, but young women seemed to suffer from it more than young men. Mr West patted her bed, after pulling up the bedclothes. 'Well, do you know you're making history with that big toe?' he said to her. It was a completely new operation.

'I'm ever so pleased with my knees,' she said, smiling gratefully to him, as if perhaps she was reserving judgement for the moment on her feet.

The next patient was also an old acquaintance. She was in her late thirties, with quite a thin and pasty face, out of proportion with the rest of her body which got bigger and bigger the further it went down into the bedclothes. Her shoulders were narrow, but her hips were immensely broad. 'Hello, my dear, you need no introduction!' he said as one of the doctors was about to present the case. 'We both know all about your case, don't we,' he said. 'I just want to have another look at your X-rays, and then I'll be back in a minute to have a talk with you.'

The group moved with the folder of X-rays to a lighted panel at the end of the ward. Once the X-rays were pinned up against the panel Mr West went over the case. 'I operated on both her hips five years ago,' he told them. 'Replaced them both. The right one has never been satisfactory from the start. She has had rashes and febrile illnesses. We asked ourselves if it was infected. Fourteen months ago we explored around that hip, but found nothing. She has a lot of sub-cutaneous fat, really a lot, and very small bones. She has very little muscle, mainly fat. I lost the femur and almost went straight through the other side without finding it. . . . The right prosthesis is still consistently painful. Look, there really is nothing at all to see on the X-rays, it's a mystery.' One of the doctors said that if anything, the left looked rather worse than the right, and the right looked very good.

'That's why I refused to touch it for a long time,' Mr West said. 'There is just a possibility that there is trouble here with the anterior wall, but it's an outside chance. We've reached the point where there's nothing else I can do but look again. She's a young woman with a family, and her walking is not good, most painful.' He shrugged his shoulders and the X-rays were unclipped as they went back to her bedside, Mr West not looking pleased with the case.

He sat down beside her bed. 'I've said it all before to you, but I just have to say it one more time,' he said. 'Your X-rays have not shown up any abnormality at all in that right hip. I cannot tell you what is the matter. I have exhausted all the things I can think of, and we've waited a long time now for it to settle itself, which it hasn't. All we can do is have a look, and maybe we'll find a piece is loose which doesn't show on the X-ray. I can't make you any promises about what the outcome will be. You know that, don't you?' She nodded. 'I must remind you,' he went on, 'that you are not in a situation where medically we have to operate. It is not a trivial procedure, and any operation carries a certain risk. Now, we could just leave it, and you could soldier on. Or else we could go ahead and operate tomorrow. It's still your choice, and you could change your mind.'

He looked at her, and she replied at once. 'That's what I want you to do, operate tomorrow.' He smiled broadly at her, rose and they moved on.

As we moved to the next room the Australian doctor talked some more about rheumatoid arthritis. 'It's a terrible disease,' he said. 'It's as bad as muscular sclerosis, except that now we can replace joints, we can mitigate its effects. Twenty-five per cent of sufferers get better, fifty per cent get it just in their bones which can be operated on to some extent, and ten per cent get it in their whole bodies, which is dreadful. Of course now almost every joint in the body can be replaced. Elbows aren't very successful yet. Yes, nearly bionic people!'

An old Maltese lady was lying with her long grey-black hair on the pillow. 'She speaks no English,' the nurse said. She was another hip fracture case.

'Get her up as soon as possible,' Mr West said. 'My Maltese is a bit rusty, so I'll just give her a wave.' He waved and stuck one thumb in the air and enunciated loudly, 'Very good!' before moving on.

The next old lady was sitting up. She had a slightly dotty air. 'You've fallen down, and had a little break in your leg. But we've fixed it all up now. All we have to do is to get you going.'

'You've finished with me?' she asked in amazement.

'Certainly. Now we just have to get you walking again.'

'OOOH!' she almost shouted with a kind of whoop. She clapped her hands above her head several times. 'I'm finished with, and I can get up!' she said.

He smiled and murmured, 'Poor dear, she doesn't know what hard work she has ahead of her,' as they moved on.

In the next bed was a diminutive old lady, exceedingly pretty, with the sort of faded blondish hair that had once been a good bright red. Mr West examined her knee, where she had had the joint replaced. 'This lady hasn't walked for five years.

185

We've replaced one knee, and soon we shall replace the other,' he said, as he gently prodded it. She looked at the other doctors nervously, but clearly had a respect verging on adoration for Mr West. He suggested they should perhaps take a swab from her wound, to check its bacteriology.

I was standing at the back of the group with the Australian. He said in a quiet voice, 'In some countries they don't bother to treat cases like hers. She was managing all right in a wheel-chair, you could say. She's elderly in her late sixties. They would give priority to the young. Well, we do give priority to people with young families, and she has been on the waiting list for five years, but now she'll be able to walk. We believe here that it's worth it.'

Another woman in her late sixties was sitting fully dressed beside her bed, her cropped iron grey hair neat. She was reading a true-story magazine called the *People's Friend* as we approached. One leg was in a surgical boot. She had had a badly infected hip, which Mr West had operated on, but it had left one leg shorter than the other. She had been in the hospital for a long time and was now reasonably well. Mr West rested both hands on the table at the end of her bed and said, 'I'm awfully sorry, my dear, this may sound a bit sudden, but I've got to find somewhere else for you to go. Do you know I have nearly 1000 ladies outside waiting to come into your bed?' The woman smiled and nodded. 'I understand that accommodation in convalescent homes which the social worker suggested doesn't appeal, is that right?' She nodded again, this time not smiling. 'I understand you'd like us to arrange for you to go to a convent for a while?' She said she would. He turned to the young doctor who was dealing with her. 'Where was she living before?'

The doctor said the name of the street near by, and added, 'Up four flights of stairs.'

Mr West gave a silent groan. He had been trying to get this woman moved for some time, but had so far been frustrated in the attempt. With such a waiting list his beds were especially precious.

Mr West turned back to her and gently asked her to show him how well she could walk. She set off, almost at a trot. Apart from the slight limp which she would always have she seemed steady and agile on her feet. 'Can we see how you manage the stairs?' he asked. The physiotherapist went with her down the passage to the staircase. The rest of us followed more slowly. Mr West turned to the doctor at his side and said with great firmness, 'Next week, when that social worker comes back, will you please tell her that we cannot extend our hospitality any longer to this lady.' The patient had become a social and not a medical case, and as from now, as he saw it, one of his precious beds was being hijacked by the social workers. He watched her get slowly and less certainly up and down the stairs, and as she descended he put his hand on her arm and pronounced, 'Absolutely marvellous! Right, I've cured that!'

They went into a small side room with a glass-panelled window, where the patient, an old lady, could look out and see all that was going on in the ward. She was being barrier-nursed as her wound had developed an infection which could have spread rapidly round the ward had she not been isolated. The Australian doctor explained, 'It's one of the main problems with surgery. Cross-infection can happen easily. We send swabs down to the labs all the time from anyone whose wound is leaking at all. At the moment they're all growing different bugs, which means that there's no cross-infection. In theory each patient should be kept in a different room as it is so important to the success of these operations that they don't get infected. Also, bugs picked up in hospital tend to be resistant, and difficult to treat.'

Mr West and his entourage then took a turn round the men's ward. It was at the end of that tour that they stopped and held a discussion, prompted by the American doctor. The last patient had been a Cypriot with foot trouble. The more they spoke to him, the more he developed other symptoms, and it became clear, in the words of the Sister as we left his bed-side that, 'That one's a nutter.'

The American doctor said, 'But so are so many of your patients. Look at them all! They're nearly all wrecks of one sort or another.'

Mr West threw his head back and laughed. He agreed that they were, on the whole, a pretty rum lot. 'It's true we have a pretty extraordinary lot of emotional and physical cases, and it makes my results on paper a lot worse than they might be. The patients' disabilities are terrible, so the results are relatively terrible! But then this is a bad area, to start with, a lot of elderly people, and on top of that, fifty per cent of my patients are sent not just from outside the Area, but from outside the Region. I get sent people no one else will operate on. I even get those ———— [a well-known Continental surgeon] won't operate on. Should I select more effectively? I could tell a lot of them to go somewhere else, and my results would look better! Should I ask how old they are, and whether they are managing perfectly well in a wheelchair already? I think I have to reject the pressures to pick out only the best pre-operative risks.' He paused for a moment, the others waiting on his every word. 'But then if the capacity of the plant is tight, as it is here, then you are forced to select to some extent.' He discussed the success rate of the Continental surgeon in rather disparaging terms. 'He gets healthy young people to start with, mostly with the same sorts of ski injuries,' he said. 'But you do know, I am sure, that the argument in favour of these poor old ladies is that if you can cure them enough for them to be able to manage their own lives at home for another four months, you've already covered the cost of the treatment.' There was some surprise at that, given the enormous cost of operating on them. 'But the cost of having them looked after full-time in institutions is phenomenal,' he said. And all those present were silenced.

As we walked down to another part of the hospital Mr West regaled the group with a recent political success he had scored, which gave him enormous pleasure. 'You remember recently Mr Callaghan signed a medical agreement with the Russians? They sent over a little girl with something the matter with her heart. We have *so* much spare capacity, our great and wonderful National Health, that we can treat the Russians too, and of course we'll send all *sorts* of problems over to them,' he said with gleeful sarcasm. 'Well, a short time ago I was telephoned by an important British government official and asked if I would treat an elderly Russian lady if they sent her over – something wrong with her hip they couldn't get right. Quick as anything I said, "Of course you wouldn't want her to come to me privately, would you?" They said immediately, "Oh no, certainly not. The whole point is that it must be done on the NHS." I said, "I see. So you wouldn't want her to queue-jump, or to be given special preferential treatment, would you?" The official said "Oh no, certainly not. Ordinary NHS treatment." I had him then. "Right," I said. "In that case send her over. She'll have to wait three to six months for her first out-patient appointment, and then she'll probably have to wait about five years for her operation." That silenced him. He said he'd have to go away and think about it. I haven't heard a word since. Privately, I think the old lady must be some important Russian official's mother, someone who doesn't trust her with any doctor in Russia who would know whose mother she was.' Everyone laughed.

It was now late. The rounds had taken a long time. Mr West had a great many patients under his care and he spent longer on each one, talking to them as well as discussing their case, than many consultants do. The group broke up and dispersed in different directions.

One afternoon a week Mr West makes a round of his private patients at The London Clinic. His association with the London Clinic is new. In the past all his private patients were treated in Fielden House, the private wing of The London Hospital, but fear of the imminent closure of private beds in National Health hospitals led him to get into a private hospital while there was still room, before the sudden rush of all the consultants who had used NHS private beds for their patients up till then.

The London Hospital charges £48·50 a day for room and meals, while The London Clinic charges £60 (£65 with bathroom) a day. 'There's no doubt that the Clinic is the better hotel,' says Mr West. 'You get better meals and all that sort of thing. It's a nicer place.'

A hip or knee replacement requires three weeks in hospital – that means a bed charge of about £1000 at The London Hospital, plus £100 or more for dressings and drugs. Mr West charges £300 (he will probably do about two private operations a week). The total cost to the patient, then, will be about £1400, for one knee or hip and double that for two, since each knee or hip has to be done separately, several weeks apart.

'I get all sorts of people as private patients. Once I had a docker who paid the whole thing down in cash. The main difference between going private and on the NHS is that the private patients have just one doctor, and that's the consultant, me. But with the NHS patients, I am head of a team, and I can't personally operate on them all. I am just left the difficult cases. The two doctors under me can do routine hips and knees just as well as I can, and if I'm ethical I wouldn't allow anyone to do an operation unless his results were as good as mine. But, you see, there will always be some people who want the boss to do it, and they're ready to pay for the privilege. It's totally understandable, but they don't get a different result. It all turns on the doctor–patient relationship. If they come and see you as a private patient and they like the look of you, they may want you, and they are prepared to make more effort to see that they get you. Of course as you get better known in the profession, you get a bigger and bigger practice. People come to you because they've heard of you. Under the NHS many patients are referred to me with a short covering note just addressed to "Dear Doctor" and they haven't a clue who they're getting.'

We were walking along Harley Street on our way to The London Clinic, while he was explaining about his private practice.

'There are other advantages too. The food is better if you go privately, and you get a single room. Yes, there are a number of single rooms anyway on most wards, but you can't be guaranteed one if you're NHS. One of the main advantages of going privately is for the busy executive. He needs to know exactly when he will be admitted to hospital so that he can make his plans around that date. On the NHS you never know when a bed might suddenly be available. It's a fringe benefit that many firms make available to their people, as it can pay off.'

He left until last, as if it was least important, the real reason why he has a large thriving private practice – the most understandable reason. 'The London Hospital's orthopaedic department is completely swamped. The East End is very bad, but it's the same all over the country. The queues and the waiting lists are quite appalling. The waiting list at the moment is three years for a woman and one year for a man. The orthopaedic beds in the district have just been increased to about 120, but that is quite insufficient. And now even those may be reduced in the new cuts. Of course many departments in the hospital have empty beds, kept for emergencies and such like, but our waiting list is far too long to ever have an empty bed.' (I never found a department with a plethora of empty beds, but every consultant believed that other people's beds in other departments were being wasted – a jealous fantasy, I think.)

'Many of my patients are not emergency cases,' he said. 'They are not going to die of their complaints, and many of them are not going to get much worse if they have to wait for treatment, but they are all of them in considerable pain. For many of them, life has become a nightmare; they are isolated, elderly, immobile, and they desperately need an operation to get them on their feet again. I can quite understand why so many people are prepared to spend their last bit of life savings on paying for the operation to be done privately, rather than having to suffer for another three years.' He paused as we came to the door of The London Clinic.

'But of course I get accused of deliberately fostering a long waiting list so as to entice patients into my private practice. . . .

Well, not me particularly, but I am part of the general accusation. Of course, it's nonsense. I'm having to turn away patients now, returning GPs' referrals at once and telling them to refer their patients elsewhere. I hate to do it, but it's kinder than making them wait here for so long.'

We went into the building. You would know this wasn't part of the NHS because of the silence and air of respect. It could be a high-class embalmer's – no clattering trolleys, no noisy boisterous porters, or chattering tongues of cleaners in a dozen underdeveloped languages. No smell of cabbage wafting down the corridors, or decrepit old ladies wrapped in rugs left nodding in their wheelchairs in the passage-way until there was room for them in the queue for the X-ray department. No crippled porters in unbuttoned uniforms trundling sheet-covered patients in zig-zags along the shiny floors. Where was the line of people with pink-, green- or buff-coloured cards waiting at a hatch for a dilatory appointments clerk? Where was the out-patients' waiting area with runny-nosed children, weary snapping, slapping mothers and fractious old men, waiting hour after hour to hear their name called? Where the distant sound of a savage old Sister barking at a student nurse, tired as the afternoon drew on? Where the clatter of mop and bucket on the stairs, the 'Out of Order' notice on the lift, the yawning volunteer in the dusty hospital shop? Was this a hospital or a Home of Rest?

It was the things that weren't there that was surprising. The place was empty, bare, deserted, silent. We ascended in the quiet lift. Down the corridors, no one was in sight, everything newly painted but sombre.

That week Mr West had only one patient in the Clinic, a middle-aged man who had had one hip replaced. He was in a very small room. After Mr West had examined him, I asked the man what he thought of the place.

'It's all right,' he said with some truculence. 'Not too bad. Mind you, I think they could do a damn sight better on the menu. I'm a hotelier and I know about these things.' He held out a copy of the day's menu. For breakfast there was anything you could think of, even kedgeree. For lunch and dinner there were nine choices each – yes, nine. 'I had the sole *bonne femme* last night. It was tolerable, but not excellent, if you know what I mean.' Mr West nodded agreement. 'Since I'm in the business I know what I'm talking about. Let me bore you with this menu again. See here, fish, brains, kidneys – a lot of people don't like those things. That only leaves six choices, doesn't it? Gammon – that's boring. Steak? I wouldn't trust it. *Coquille St Jacques?* A bit rich.' He put the menu down on the table beside his bed. 'Still, all in all you know, Mr West, it's not too bad in here.'

On the way out Mr West showed me one of the suites. It had a big hall-way, with a door leading into an enormous bedroom. The room was quite pretty, like a nice hotel room, with a big dressing table flounced and frilled. There was carpet on the floor, and ordinary non-hospital furniture. It was an odd place, it gave me an odd sensation. It had nothing whatever to do with a hospital. We accept so readily our only experiences of things. Hospitals are places with grim iron beds, bleak rooms and cold floors, high ceilings and unfriendly hygiene. Was all that due to lack of money? Could hospitals be made to look a little more like homes? If the most expensive suite has a carpet and ordinary furniture, it can't be considerations of hygiene that make hospitals bare and cold, it must be money. There was a sitting-room too, with a spare bed for visitors, and a writing table; a bright blue bathroom was through another door.

We walked through the building and out of another door, over to a block in Harley Street where Mr West was to hold his private out-patients clinic that afternoon.

Harley Street is owned almost entirely by one property concern, the Howard De Walden Estate. They lay down strict rules. One of the rules is that no consulting rooms are to be let out by the day, or half-day to doctors. One doctor must rent one room for the whole week. This building was one of the very few not owned by the company, and Mr West rented a consulting room and a receptionist for one afternoon a week.

Mr West paid £300 a year for the half-day and receptionist. He usually fitted in about six or more patients. He spent three-quarters of an hour on a new patient, and half an hour on an old one – longer than the average NHS out-patient appointment. He said most of his patients were English, though on this occasion three were foreign.

The consulting room and reception area were modern crisp and elegant. No one was waiting, as the appointments system was carefully worked out as it is in the NHS – but since there are so few private patients, the timing can be kept to. Mr West treated his patients with great politeness. He rose from his chair to greet them when they came into the room. The receptionist actually ushered them in, to get them over that sticky moment of coming into a doctor's surgery. He helped the ladies out of their coats, which he thoughtfully hung up for them. In short, the patients were treated with the sort of deference money can buy in a hairdresser's, a department store or a restaurant, but which the NHS often seems to have failed to purchase for its clients.

The first person on the list was a Canadian woman, mother of a fourteen-year-old boy who suffered from a rare affliction of the knee-caps which sometimes assails adolescents. She came alone, as she happened to be passing through London. Mr West had operated on the boy once, a small operation with only a sixty to seventy per cent chance of success. He said the boy was spoiled and over-cared for. But he was patient with the mother as the story rambled on. It appeared that he had sent them back after the operation with firm instructions.

'You stressed – no more operations, no more treatment, and told us not to say a word about his knees any more – and I promise you we never mentioned them at all. But then he started saying they were hurting and swelling.'

'Was the swelling visible to you?' he asked.

'Oh yes. And then the specialist back home put him back in plaster and it didn't help. Then he wanted to do a re-alignment. I couldn't stop them. I had to do something. The scars were very neat, but the pain and swelling was not affected. Now they're talking about removing his knee-caps, and I want your opinion on that? Another doctor told me it would be a disaster.'

'Well, it's not a very serious thing, but it's not advisable. I didn't say he was making a thing out of it deliberately, but I suggested you try not to force his attention on to his knees.'

'Oh but we don't. . . .'

The discussion rambled on for a long time, mostly with the woman talking and Mr West making polite but firm interjections.

'The hardest advice to follow is to sit tight and endure it. For the next four or five years soldier on, no plaster, no operations, no stairs, no swimming.'

She was grateful, but perhaps not convinced. He helped her into her coat, she took up her shopping bags and left. Mr West doubted that much notice would be taken of his advice.

The next patient was a young plain girl from the Middle East who walked with a bad limp. She had her young cousin with her, who acted as interpreter. 'I occasionally get these people,' Mr West said. 'All civil servants in her country have the right to get the government to pay for their treatment in England, if there aren't proper facilities there for them. It's all paid for through their consulate.'

Later I was talking with some journalist friends from this girl's country, and they said that in fact that was not exactly the system. Civil servants did not have the right to get free treatment here, nor did anyone else. But if you knew someone, who knew someone, it was sometimes something that could be fixed. Often, in fact usually, the illness could be treated in that country's hospitals; sometimes people came over for treatment who were not ill at all, but wanting a holiday. They also averred that some unscrupulous British consultants were to be found around the Middle East touting for business, and waving glossy brochures for such luxury hospitals like the new Cavendish and Wellington.

The truth of this is, of course, uncheckable, but they said there was great indignation at home about this particular form of nepotism and corruption. It is regarded as a wicked drain on their currency and in an underdeveloped country, an out-rageously misplaced use of medical funds.

However, this girl, who was apparently not rich, well educated or well connected, was desperately in need. How she had managed to pull off the free treatment wasn't clear.

The first thing Mr West did was to clear up the situation with the consulate, whom he should write to in their medical section, etc.

'Now, what's the problem?' he asked, pressing his finger tips together, that well-known professional mannerism.

The girl handed over a letter, creased and ragged. 'This is doctor at home writes,' said her cousin. He perused the document. It explained that the girl was born with trouble in both hips and that she wants to get married. She wants the function in both hips improved.

'What does she want? Relief from pain?' he asked.

'Yes, the pain,' said the cousin. The girl was nodding and clearly understood a little English.

'How far can she walk?' he asked.

The two girls consulted for a moment. 'She say five to ten minutes. Sometimes she catches and stops.'

'Then she waits for the pain to stop and walks on?'

'Yes.'

'Does she get pain at night?' More consultation.

'When she turns over.'

'Can she touch her feet?'

'Only when she sits down. She can hardly separate her legs. She wants to get married,' said the cousin.

'How would she feel if I said I could relieve all the pain but not improve the movement at all?'

'Please. . . . I don't want to say that to her. Be too disappointed. She has been told she can never get married or have babies.'

'She could get married, as she is,' he answered, 'though it might not be very satisfactory. She could have babies by caesarean section.' The cousin looked blank, not as though she hadn't understood, but as though she was going to hold out

196

for something better, and she didn't translate any of this. Mr West asked the girl to go into the next room and take her clothes off. The two went in together.

'The trouble with having an international practice,' Mr West said to me while he was waiting for her to get ready, 'is that you can't follow up on your cases. This girl is something of a curiosity. You'd never find a person of her age here with this complaint. It would have been put right soon after birth. It's very unusual to have to replace both hips at the age of twenty-eight. Of course I've never been to the Middle East so I don't know much about their culture, but I understand that to be unmarried there is an absolute disaster for a girl. Unmarried girls just perish, become paupers.'

The cousin came back into the room and sat down again.

'Does she have a fiancé now?' he asked her.

'No. She had one a long time ago. But she gave him up when they told her the hips would not be better.'

Mr West went in to examine her. It didn't take very long, and simply confirmed the diagnosis already made on her. When he came back, and washed his hands at the basin he said thoughtfully. 'Yes, the legs are very stiff and straight, and there is very little movement in the hip. To an English spinster I might suggest something else, but for an unmarried Middle Eastern girl . . .' He came back to his desk and sat down. He wrote out a form ordering an X-ray to be done, while he was waiting for the girl to get dressed.

'Well,' he said to them both when they were seated before him again, 'your cousin has stiff and painful hips. She will not die, as she is. It will not spread to other joints. But it is a disease that may get a bit worse, hurt a bit more and become stiffer. This is not something she must suffer. But she must weigh all the advantages and disadvantages. Now, will you tell her that much first?' He waited while the cousin translated.

'All right?' he asked when she had stopped. 'There is only one operation that will both get rid of the pain and increase the movement. There is another operation that will just relieve the pain. Is it essential to get movement? I think she'll say it is, but I want to hear it from her before we proceed.'

'She need the both of it,' said the cousin. 'But the pain the most.'

'The operation, then, will give movement as well, if successful, and it will get rid of all the pain. She will be able to move much more, to lift her legs, and part them much more. She will be able to have sexual intercourse and babies. But she will still not be completely normal. Does she know that I could advise her on how, without any operation, she could have sexual intercourse in a way that her hips could manage? I want to be sure she really understands the point of this operation.'

'She says she wants her hips better.'

'Well, the pain will go. . . .'

'Good!' the girl herself suddenly said.

'Now the bad news. And it is very important she understands. She could end up worse than she is now. If the joint had to be removed for any reason one leg could end up shorter than the other. She could have more movement but less strength. No operation is guaranteed. No operation cannot go wrong. There is a one or two in a hundred chance that it will go wrong. If she was sixty, no problem, I wouldn't hesitate to do it. But at her age that new joint is going to have to last fifty or sixty years, and so far they've only been inside people for a few years and we don't know how they last. It may come loose and need operating on again some time. Do you know you could get here for that? The wound can become infected and then we might have to take it out. I'm putting it at its worst so you understand. All these risks together are one or two in a hundred. She could have nothing done. Or she could have a much simpler operation to stiffen the joints, relieving the pain but giving no more movement. Tell her all that.'

It took a suspiciously short time for that to be explained. It sounded like less than one sentence. 'God knows what she's getting,' Mr West muttered half under his breath.

'She say she don't mind if she go home in a wheel-chair.

At least she will have tried. She say it doesn't matter about the babies. She wants to be married. She say too that she could have had the operation when she was four, but her mother would not allow it.'

'Well, tell her not to be sorry about that any more. An end is in sight. Bring her to the hospital at four-thirty on Sunday and I will operate on Monday morning.'

Full of gratitude, the girl close to tears, they made their way out of the room.

Mr West set about putting his consulting room to rights. He straightened the blankets on the examining couch next door, and stretched a new piece of blue paper sheeting across it – a curious sight to see a consultant happily doing a nurse's job.

There followed a nice district nurse in her sixties from Wales whose knee was incapacitating her in her travels round the wild countryside. She looked after her elderly mother, had no money except her life savings, and was coming privately, because if she had to wait for treatment on the National Health her loss of earnings while she wasn't working would be a more crippling expense than the cost of the private operation. She knew that on the National Health she would have to wait perhaps three or more years.

Mr West was gentle and sympathetic. He didn't like to take her life's savings, so he decided to fiddle his waiting list, and put her very near the top, on the National Health. I don't know if she quite realized what he was doing. She may have thought that going as a private patient for a consultation could always mean jumping the waiting list as a National Health patient, which it certainly doesn't. In the event, she was treated privately and the cost was covered by an organization.

There followed two more routine knee cases, one a middle-aged woman who ran a boarding house and had a little money saved, the other a businessman. The last patient of the day was the sort of difficult case grumbled about on every ward. Perhaps he was worse for being a private patient – eager to make sure he squeezed his last pennyworth out of the doctor. But probably he would have been as bad on the NHS, full of all the self-righteousness of the life-long taxpayer. However his money had probably bought him a little more patience than he would have met with elsewhere, and Mr West was remarkably patient, though occasionally he could be seen bubbling beneath the skin.

Mr Walsh came into the room with a curious gnomish caper, like a ferociously angry Rumpelstiltskin – tiny, crumpled with a sour-looking mouth.

'You have no letter of referral?' asked Mr West, somewhat timidly confronting the seething aggression flooding across the desk from his patient.

'No,' was the answer. 'I came to you because I know a lot about medical things, and my informants in high places tell me you are the best man for my complaint. Also, I heard you on the radio last week.' Mr West suppressed a smile.

'What seems to be the trouble?'

'I've been arthritic for many years, mainly in the knee. Now it's gone to the ankles and some finger joints. I suppose it's in the spine at the base of the vertebrae,' he added jutting his chin a little as if defying any challenge to his superior knowledge.

'How are your hips?'

'I felt it in the left hip last year but it's eased up.'

'I see,' said Mr West taking notes.

'I believe I have osteo not rheumatoid, from what I've read,' Mr Walsh challenged again.

'Which joint would you say gave you the most trouble?' Mr West asked.

Mr Walsh answered the question in a comically roundabout way. 'I believe you have originated or at least become proficient in operations on new knee joints. I contacted another orthopaedic surgeon and he thought you were the best.'

'So your problem is your knee?'

'Well my ankle is badly thickened, but let's deal with the knee first, shall we?' He spoke as if he wanted to buy the joint that the doctor was best at rather than the joint he most needed, like choosing the chef's speciality from the menu.

'Mr Walsh,' said Mr West, trying for the first time to take an authoritative hold on the conversation, 'I need to know what is the major problem in your legs.'

'The knee joints,' he spat out, like bullets from an automatic.

'Is one worse than the other?'

'The left is worse. The quadricep muscles are much worse and my right ankle is worse due to arthritic growth.'

Mr West consistently disregarded the patient's medical jargon.

'All right, lets start again. How do you go downstairs?'

'My left knee hasn't got the flexibility of my right one, but it's not a good ankle. I go right foot first.'

'How far can you walk?'

'Oh I do walk, doctor. I believe in keeping mobile. I walk a few miles.'

'A few miles! I don't get many people here who can do that!'

'But the walking is very restricted. I used to go much further and when I'm sitting down I'm loath to get up. I go for a good walk in the park on Sunday though.'

'So you're not much restricted?'

'Yes I am. What is your specific question?'

'When you go for a walk are you stopped by the pain, yes or no?' Mr West's voice rose and was not far from a shout.

'No,' was the surprising answer.

'Right, your walking then is not restricted.'

'It is. I go by bus and Tube mostly when I used always to walk.'

Mr West counted to ten before asking Mr Walsh to go into the next room, remove his trousers and sit on the bed for examination.

The conversation continued through the door.

'Are you awoken at night by the pain?'

'No.'

'Does this hurt? Does this? Or this?'

'The pain here is not comparable to there. My legs are bowed as you'll observe.'

Eventually they were agreed that his left knee and right

ankle were not good. Mr West came back to his consulting room looking, for him, rather ruffled and cross. Mr Walsh followed shortly, all his defences up.

'Will you X-ray me all over?' he asked.

'Just the left knee. Are those some X-rays you've got with you?' he asked as the patient pulled out a large folder.

'They're just of my spine, but I thought they might interest you.'

'I don't think I need to look at your spine. It's the knee. You have got some osteo arthritis, Mr Walsh. The joints have become hard and stiff. . . .'

'Oh I know all that! I have no sinovial fluid in the knee.'

Mr West took another deep breath and continued as if uninterrupted.

'There are three options. You could do nothing at all about it. The pain could get worse but it might not. You could have the operation done at some future date when it seemed to you absolutely essential. Or you could have it done now. I would replace the surfaces of your bones but leave the knee cap. You might still get some discomfort, the odd twinge, but the pain when walking would go.'

'Is it safe?'

'No operation at sixty-seven is entirely safe,' Mr West said, perhaps enjoying spelling out the danger. 'But this one isn't especially dangerous. It could go wrong and you might end up having to have the leg stiffened, though it's unlikely.'

'Well, if all goes well, I think I'll have the other one done too.'

He then pondered on when to have it done and they agreed a date. He rose to leave the room, and Mr West rose too, anxious to be rid of him.

'There's just one thing though,' said the patient. 'I was under the impression you used a ferrous substance.'

'I do, metal on plastic.'

'Is it an alloy?'

'I use cobalt, chrome and polyethylene.'

'Is there a coating over the metal?'

'No.'

'It's a ball and socket joint?'

'Yes.'

'It really works without a coating?'

'YES.'

'It really will fit me nicely? The knee isn't a simple structure to mess around with you know?'

'I KNOW!'

'Is our interview terminated now?'

'YES! It is! Good-bye!'

'One has to be certain about these things. Good-bye,' and he finally went out of the room.

'Jesus Christ!' Mr West shouted, hardly before the door had closed. It was an uncharacteristic outburst. Normally he is utterly composed. In the event, he refused to operate on this man.

7

Kidneys

In the Sisters' dining-room one of the nurses from the operating theatres was grumbling, 'I've got Frankenstein this afternoon.' She was talking about Dr Frank Goodwin, consultant nephrologist, kidney specialist. As she hurried away I didn't have time to ask why she gave him that name. Just because he was called Frank? Or on account of the Frankensteinian side of kidney transplants? Slight, with dapper good dark looks, he had bright glittery eyes. He looked and was more than a little obsessional. He worked relentlessly and was surprised and uncomprehending of anything less than total dedication in those under him. He gave the nurses a hard time. The patients had a devoted faith in him, and were awed and abashed, in spite of his slightly strained attempts at being relaxed with them. His dealings with the Administrators and others in the hospital were not always easy; when he was angry, people kept out of his way.

Dr Goodwin set up the dialysis (kidney-machine) unit almost single-handed. Kidney machines had been invented some years previously though there were very few in existence, when a local GP fell ill with kidney failure. Dr Goodwin built a machine himself, and saved his colleague's life. After this success The London Hospital was given the money to set up the Hanbury Dialysis Unit.

There is something that grabs the imagination about kidney machines. In America kidney-machine patients are the only non-welfare cases to receive state grants – the other chronic illnesses have to fend for themselves. In England too, it is fairly easy for someone who requires a kidney machine to be rehoused, and to have his new house properly adapted at the hospital's expense, while people with other disabilities get short shrift.

Perhaps it was the early rumours about kidney machines that gave kidney diseases special status. In early days of dialysis no doctor envisaged that a patient would ever be able to have a machine at home and learn to use it himself. It is a very dangerous and complicated business. It was assumed that all patients would have to come into hospital three times a week to be dialysed by nurses, and that there would never be the beds or the money for all those suffering from kidney failure to be treated this way. Once it was realized that people could be trained to do it themselves, that it was only the capital cost of the machines, and the outlay for servicing them involved, everyone breathed a sigh of relief, and dialysis units were set up throughout the country by the Ministry of Health. It costs about £4500 to set up a machine at home, and at The London the only criterion is whether a person will manage and thrive on kidney dialysis at home. But the UK is low on the list of people per million receiving dialysis or transplant, compared with the rest of Europe. Outside London treatment is not so readily available.

The London Hospital's Dialysis Unit is separate and sealed off from the rest of the hospital, a sterile zone, with warning signs outside telling people not to come in. At one end is the ward of nine beds, with nine machines, nine artificial kidneys, and nine patients, wired up to them, looking blank and distant amongst that roomful of dials, with bright red tubes full of blood weaving in and out. There is a hum of the pumps, a constant sound in your ears that deadens the noise of voices, and makes each patient seem remote on his island amongst all this hardware. It reminded me of an open-plan office, with the machines dividing up the room like filing cabinets, only instead of desks and telephone wires, there were beds and tubes.

Willy Stephens was a new patient. He was still in his first

few weeks on a machine. There was much discussion about him at dialysis team meetings, as there is always about someone just starting on the long road to dialysing at home. The staff had thought he would do very well with the training, being bright and energetic. Alan Hawkes, the chief technician, said he usually knew who would be a quick learner and he had picked out Willy as he'd shown interest and had asked all the right questions in the first few sessions.

Since then, though, they had been a little disappointed with his progress, and he seemed to have sensed this. Ros Levenson, the social worker, said he was having particular trouble acknowledging to himself that he was seriously ill; he was resisting the training. She reported that he was refusing to take time off work, although he easily could, and that he had suddenly started an absurdly energetic redecorating of his house from top to bottom. This, she said, was part of his denial that he was ill, and it left him so exhausted that he couldn't concentrate on learning how to use the machine. Also, she said, he hated to feel he was being talked about all the time by the team, and discussed in case conferences.

Willy Stephens was a man in his early thirties, married with several young children. When I met him in the unit he was the only patient being dialysed from a chair, and not lying on a bed – perhaps another way of trying to pretend to himself that dialysis wasn't important. He was very yellow faced, and had heavily nicotine-stained fingers. His manner was jovial, talkative, forthright but a little forced, as if he was continually studying himself from outside to check that he was putting up a good performance.

'Oh, it's not too hard to learn,' he said breezily, lighting a cigarette straight after having put one out. 'But to tell the truth the circumstances in this place make it hard. My head feels terrible from the lack of ventilation. I keep asking them to open a window, but they won't. It keeps me awake, I find, to sit in a chair.

'The first day I came in here I was stunned. I'd just never seen anything like it. I think it was all this tubing. I thought at first it was red tubing. I didn't realize it was transparent and the red was the blood. At first the nurses do absolutely everything for you, but then they make you start to do some of it yourself. That's when it really dawns on you what it's all about.'

He seemed to know what was being said about him as he said right away, 'I find it hard to call myself ill. Right up until just a month or two ago I was playing rugby all the time, not a care in the world – I was perfectly well. It happened one afternoon when I was going to work. I got to Aldgate station and I came over funny. I felt a terrible pounding in the chest and all leaden-legged. When I got into work I went to the doctor there and he checked me over. He couldn't find anything wrong. He even said as a joke that he'd sign a life insurance policy for me any time I liked!

'Then the same thing happened again the next day – oddly enough in the same place, at the station, and I went back to the doctor. This time he did a urine test on me. Then he told me I had to go straight to hospital, right away, not even time to go home and get my things. By that time I was feeling perfectly fit again, and I thought there was nothing the matter.

'When I got here the Registrar said I had to go straight to bed. I said, "I can't, not now. I've got my work to do, and I've got to go home. I just had a temporary attack." He said I'd have to stay three or four days for some tests, but I stayed a month. I felt so well that I thought the doctors were just experimenting with me. I kept asking, "Are you sure I have to stay in?" I used to run all the errands and carry all the messages in the ward. I was dancing around, I was the fittest one there. But it was only when I came out of hospital that I realized how weak I was compared to normal people.

'In hospital if I saw or smelt anything that was even just a little bit nasty, I'd retch. The nurses said that kidney patients are known for that. But I've got over it now, mostly.

'The first day they put me on the machine for three hours. I've never had such a head-ache in my life. But I must admit, the next day I felt fantastic.

'But I won't change my life just for the machine. I'm much

too busy. I'm really looking forward to going home. I've got the confidence to manage this at home now. My wife is so good and calm. She'll cope. Luckily we've got a very big house and there'll be plenty of room for the thing. I would have despaired if we'd had to move. I really love the house.'

He paused to light another cigarette and then stared up at the machine from his low armchair. 'It's a very strange thing, digging needles into yourself, when you stop and think about it. It's quite unnatural and it goes against everything your body tells you is right. The needling is terrible. I've got a tough skin, and I have to try and sort of screw it in. The nurses tell you to push it in, but it won't go unless I screw it hard as well. I've been in the East and my skin has been baked hard in the sun and it's tough,' he said, rubbing his arm.

'I'm often depressed. Perhaps because I'm living so near the brink. It isn't nice to think there is only that supporting me,' and he gave the machine a sour look. 'Sometimes I don't want to live,' he said, and broke into a fit of coughing, after which he stubbed out his cigarette, half-smoked. 'But then you think of your family. Probably otherwise I wouldn't . . . you know, go on with the thing, in periods of depression. What's the use, I ask myself, and so on.' Then he seemed to feel he was slipping and he pulled himself together and shifted his position in his chair.

'I've changed a lot in this very short time. I used to be irritable – oh, with everything, my wife, the children and so on, but not now. Other patients say the same thing. Is it the fear of dying or is it something chemical? . . . But the one thing I can't stand is the diet. Vegetables twice cooked, and only six cups of liquid a day.

'You know, I used to love drinking ice-cold milk. Sometimes in one day I'd drink three pints of it, straight from the fridge, so you can imagine how I suffer on so little to drink. Now, if you drink more than you're supposed to it's like pouring liquid into your socks. It just stays there and doesn't disperse.'

He reached for another cigarette and saw me glance at his

ash tray, full to the brim with ash and ends. 'I smoke twice as many when I'm in hospital as I do at any other time. . . . It's the tension and the boredom and the being forced to sit still so long. If you're an active man like me, it's like being chained up. I smoke more than forty when I'm on the machine.'

He paused while he slowly uncrossed his legs that were resting on another chair. 'They've never suggested my having a transplant. I suppose you have to ask specially for one. I'm afraid of having one anyway. I had a bad experience in the ward. There was a chap in the next bed to me, just the same age, and lived near me. Our wives knew each other, used the same shop, though I didn't know the family. Well, he went into the operating theatre one day for a transplant, and he died. They didn't tell me at the time, when I asked how he was doing. I got a shock when I found out, and it scared me badly. Of course the doctors all said not to worry, and what I'd got wasn't at all the same disease he had. But all the same, it gave me a nasty turn, and I'm not that gone on transplants now. . . . Of course maybe later on, I might consider it, in a few years or so.'

Taking another cigarette he drew deeply on it and said, 'I'm really not like this at all. I'm a different man usually. In here I'm full of a lot of verbal banter with the nurses and so on, jolly and full of jokes. I don't know why. I'm not a bit like that at home or at work. Perhaps it's a defence against the machine, do you think? . . . You know, if someone had told me years ago that I'd be on a machine I'd have said, "NO, not on your life. I'd rather die." But here I am, aren't I? At least at the moment. But you know, I'm sure there are plenty of people who just can't accept it, when it comes to it.

'Of course, the doctors and nurses wouldn't tell you about it, but I've heard things, and I understand. It would be so easy to despair. You could do things – just give up. Maybe it would look like an accident, maybe it would be half an accident. One night, the lines from the machine come apart while you're dozing, and the blood runs out and you just bleed to death quietly. It's an easy suicide. If you think about it, it's not even a suicide. It's just letting things be . . . letting nature take its course. I can't help admitting there is always that in your mind — must be the same with all of us, on bad days.'

One afternoon, Ros Levenson, the nephrology department social worker, took me on a visit to one of her home dialysis patients. All the patients on the ward went home as soon as they were trained.

She paid regular visits to the patients on machines to see how they were managing.

'To be quite frank,' she said, 'This couple are something of a miracle. We never thought they'd learn. Some of the team were against even trying with them, but, somehow or other, here they are, still at it, even though I don't think they manage very well.'

Norman and Irene live in a small terraced house not far from the hospital. They were rehoused from the next-door borough of Bethnal Green when Norman had to go onto a kidney machine.

We knocked on the front door and Irene opened it after a short pause. She had been warned of our visit. Ros knows all her patients well and they are glad to see her. Irene smiled and showed us in. There was a smell of mutton cooking, and Ros said it smelled good. Irene apologized for her slippers. 'Norman's in bed, I'm afraid, but he'll be down shortly. It's not one of his good days, I'm afraid.'

She led us into the kitchen and made a pot of tea. 'We've had a lot more trouble with the benefit,' she said to Ros as she put the pot down on the table. She looked tired and not very strong, but she was a cheerful woman, underneath. She took a sheaf of official forms and papers down from the mantelpiece for Ros to sort out. She looked through them and said, 'I'm sorry it's all so difficult, Irene. Let me take these away with me and see what I can do.'

Norman came downstairs, buttoning a clean shirt, his feet shuffling a bit in his slippers. He gave a smile and a firm handshake. 'Sorry not to have been here, Ros, but to tell the truth, I'm not so good today,' He had a very deep growly voice, and he sat himself down beside the gas fire. 'How's everyone?' he asked. 'Been any transplants this week?' Ros said there hadn't.

Norman began talking about himself. 'I can tell you, when I saw the thing I thought we'd never get the hang of it. No, it didn't exactly frighten us though, as we'd seen one before. A man in our road, a Polish man, had one, though we never took much notice of it. The artificial kidney itself was no problem, it was the machine and all the clocks on it. But you just learn one part of it at a time, and there was no day you didn't learn something, what the alarms are all for, for example, and how to turn them off yourself. You learn which one is for a blood leak, which for high pressure, or for low pressure. But I was confident enough by the time I came home. I was longer learning than most patients, mind you. One reason was that we had to wait twelve months to get rehoused. We had a nice place in Bethnal Green, but with only three bedrooms and we have three kids. They offered us another place soon but it was no bigger so we turned it down. You see you need a whole room for the machine.'

'It's a very nice house we have here,' Irene said. 'It's nice to have a garden. It gives him something to do with his time.'

'But I minded having to leave Bethnal Green,' said Norman. 'We both lived there all our lives and we don't know anybody here. We have no friends. I know it isn't far away, but I never have the energy to go there on the bus. All my friends are in the pub over there, and I can't seem to have the strength to go on the bus. I don't have the heart. I did go to Bethnal Green for a funeral last week, for two hours, and that was nice. I saw my friends then.'

'Yes, we had a very nice time, though it was only a couple of hours. It was an outing,' Irene said.

'Every Monday is the worst for me. I don't know why. I feel really fagged out on Mondays. . . . Oh yes, you could say my life has changed a lot. I used to like to go out, but we have no night life now. I hardly set foot outside the door. Thank goodness for the television.' He paused, looking down at the fire.

You can't ever really plan anything. You have to learn to make use of your good days. You learn to say, "This is a good day, I'll do it today."'

Irene said, 'A nice girl offered to take us to the seaside for the day not long ago, and we had it all set up in advance. But when the day came he wasn't feeling good and he felt bad in that van, and he vomited a lot. You can't plan, like he says.' She paused. 'Then there was the day your sister came all the way from Ireland to see you and something went wrong and you had to go in the hospital. Oh, it's not a real life at all that he leads. The man's alive, and that's about all you can say about him, isn't that right, Norman?'

'It's no sort of life,' he agreed, reaching for a cigarette. 'Then people give you funny looks when you tell them about the machine. Maybe they get the idea you aren't human. You're a sort of Frankenstein perhaps. A neighbour asked the other day if I have to lie down on top of the machine, like recharging a battery I suppose. My sister came and watched me go on the machine one night, and she saw it, the needling and all, but her husband wouldn't go in the room.'

I asked what their children thought of it. They had two sons, one at work, one in college, and a daughter still at school.

'They don't want to know,' Norman said sadly. 'They don't want to know nothing about it, or to hear nothing about it. If I'm all right, then they're all right. But it's happened a couple of times when I've been needling myself I've missed the vein, and I've had to call one of them to fetch another needle. They don't like it.'

'Well, you can't expect them to do things for you,' Irene said.

'But I thought they might learn to help, and that, but, well, kids today . . . ' Norman said.

'Of course Nora [another patient], her boy used to do everything for her, didn't he?' Irene said. 'I used to tell them to learn it, but they're not interested. By the way,' she said suddenly changing the subject, 'How's that woman, I forget her name, that German woman?'

'I'm afraid she died a few days ago,' Ros answered boldly.

Irene made a small sudden gesture, as if to cross herself. 'It's a mercy! Thank God! He has taken his own. She wasn't for this world you know. Thanks for the mercy of God! And the young girl, Linda, how's she doing?'

'Fine, she's just fine,' Ros said.

'Well,' Norman said to me, getting slowly to his feet and putting his tea cup back on the table. 'Would you like to see the machine upstairs? I'll explain how it works.'

They ushered me upstairs to the special room. It was covered in bright yellow flowery wallpaper. She saw me looking at it. 'Yes, they do it all up for you, you know. The hospital fitters do it all.'

It was a small room next door to their bedroom. A big iron hospital bed took up most of the space. Above the bed was a string with an alarm, and next to it was the machine, tall and glittery with its clocks and dials. A large sluice-type sink had been plumbed into one corner of the room, and the big artificial kidney stood beside it. Stacked in the corners and in the cupboards of the room were huge cardboard boxes full of new supplies – needles, tubes, bowls, cotton wool, canisters of dialysing fluid for the kidney. It was quite a formidable sight; the gayness of the yellow flowers on the wall was no match for the starkness of the machine and the medical supplies.

Norman lay down on the bed with his arm outstretched and began to explain how he fixed himself onto it. 'The needling is the bad job,' he said, holding up one of the huge needles. 'Sometimes you get vein collapse and you have to sit for half an hour with a hot pad on your arm. I'm afraid this dial here has got a bit messy,' he said pointing to a glass panel on the machine. 'The lines came apart the other day and blood splattered all over the place. How it got inside this dial, I don't know. Of course I always do the needling myself. Some patients have their husbands or wives do it, but I'd never trust Irene.'

'Oh no, I'd never do it, never,' Irene said with a shudder from the doorway. She began pointing out the different supplies. 'I must admit, it always seems a waste to me to have to throw all this tubing away after each session. You'd think they'd sterilize it and use it again, wouldn't you? I don't like to think what it costs the taxpayer.'

'Well, you have to be sure, don't you?' Norman said. 'My life depends on it. You know the other day the pump on the machine broke down while I was dialysing. Irene ran to the phone and the technician jumped in his van to come and fix it. Irene had to put all these tubes full of blood into buckets of warm water, while it wasn't circulating and was out of my body. They look a bit nasty, don't they, these transparent tubes when they're full of blood?'

Irene and Norman looked with some awe at this heap of equipment that had found its way into their lives. They approached the room with reverence – it was the tabernacle of the house. Irene explained how often she cleaned and scrubbed everything in it. Yet they didn't seem to be at ease, or to have assimilated the contents of that room into their possessions. They didn't seem to feel it belonged to them. They looked, as they stood in the doorway, like two small birds contemplating with puzzlement a monstrous and demanding cuckoo that had found its way into their nest.

It takes half an hour to set up the machine, ready for dialysing. It is connected to the artificial kidney which looks like a huge white screen on a hinge. The blood is pumped out of the arm into the kidney, which is like a giant filter paper, and then back into the body. Once the machine is operating fully, about a pint of blood at a time is outside the body.

The needling is much the worst part of it, according to the patients I spoke to. It is no ordinary needle but a very large one indeed, about an inch of which is passed into the vein after a local anaesthetic has been injected in the skin. Most of the dialysis patients have to undergo a special operation to make a 'fistula', an enlargement of the veins in one arm to make this easier. When you put a hand on one of these arms with enlarged veins you can feel, almost hear the gushing of the blood, the pulse is so strong. The needle usually takes time to insert, and often it is very difficult to get in right, with a fast enough flow of blood pumping into the machine. Sometimes they have to try over and over again and it can be painful and upsetting.

The patient, once plugged into the machine, lies on the bed for seven hours dozing lightly, if he's lucky. Many patients sleep well but some say they can't sleep on the machine at all. Alarms ring if anything goes wrong, and a buzzer is put into the room so that the other person in the house can be called for help.

All the dialysis patients from the hospital have to go on to their machines on the same three evenings, when there is an emergency service operating. Technicians in vans stand by on three nights a week to dash to the scene if someone's machine breaks down, or leaks.

It takes an hour and a half to clean out the machine after use each time, so the whole operation takes about nine to ten hours. Once a week, usually on Saturdays, the artificial kidney has to be stripped and rebuilt. It needs two people to do this and takes three hours, so the kidney machine patient can reckon on three nights sometimes with little sleep, and Saturday mornings, devoted to it. It is easy to see why so many of them find it hard to lead normal lives.

All patients on machines have to go on to a strict diet for the rest of their lives. The diet is carefully balanced to minimize certain chemicals that accumulate in the body in renal failure. In some patients only a pint of liquid each day in any form is allowed. All vegetables have to be cooked for a long time to reduce their potassium content, very little chocolate is allowed, and not much salt. The whole intake of food has to be scientifically calculated. It is, as the dietician stressed, quite adequate, and sustaining. The patients complain most about the lack of liquid.

The patients have to go for regular blood tests, and from the results the dieticians can tell at once how well they have been keeping to the diet. The real killer is potassium. Too much potassium causes instant heart attacks in kidney patients, with no warning symptoms. The doctors can tell something about a patient's mental state from how well he keeps to the diet. It is well known amongst them that some patients can lose heart and quietly commit suicide by ceasing to care and take precautions. Some patients on machines die because consciously or not quite consciously they have decided not to go on fighting, overwhelmed by the fact that there is no hope that things will improve.

Some patients, however, do well and one afternoon, in the dialysis out-patients' clinic, I did see one man who was a model patient. He even looked quite well, for a dialysis patient. He and his wife bounced into the room, beaming and keen to tell how well he was. He went ski-ing, surfing, climbing, and hiking.

The doctor took him through the questionnaire, almost as a matter of form. His potassium was up, but his fistula was in good order. 'My wife needles. I used to but it took too long,' he said. He was a busy local council officer in his early thirties. 'The only thing I suffer from is shortage of sleep,' he said. Did he take any pills? 'Only half a mogadon if the needling is going badly. . . .' How was he managing on the diet? His wife answered, 'He does all his own cooking. He won't let me near his food. He makes all these elaborate exotic things for himself.' What about transplantation? (This was asked of all kidney patients every three months.) 'No, thank you,' he said politely, as if he'd been offered a sugar bun.

'We rebuild the kidney on Tuesdays instead of Saturdays so as to get an unbroken weekend for going away in our caravan,' he was explaining. 'What did I think of it at first? Well, I just said to myself, if so many other people have got used to it as a way of life there's no reason why I shouldn't. I hated it in hospital. When you're inside, the machine is all you're thinking about. But once you get it home it just merges into the rest of your normal life.'

The doctor asked the wife how she was managing. 'Well, I think I'd find it easier if I had kids. Then I'd be at home all day.

But as I'm working it's a bit tough to have housework, job and the machine to cope with.'

Everyone was pleased with this couple. Even the doctors and nurses were surprised by them.

The next morning there was a meeting to discuss the progress and condition of the home dialysis patients. At the meeting doctors, social workers, dieticians and technicians discussed how each patient was getting along. Results of analyses of blood and of dialysis fluid were scrutinized to see that dialysis was proceeding satisfactorily. Regular X-rays of the bones were also taken. Vitamin D, deficiency of which causes rickets, can only be effective in the body if the kidneys are working properly, so those without kidneys tend to suffer from bone disease.

The patients were all well known to everyone at the meeting. They had, after all, spent many months in the unit being trained to use their machines, and many of them had now been dialysing at home for several years.

A sixteen-year-old girl was doing well, with her father needling her, no problem. A middle-aged woman was showing definite signs of bone erosion in her hands, on the X-ray. She complained her husband never got any sleep. 'He's in a panic,' the social worker said. 'It's a miracle he copes at all.' A West Indian woman wanted to be admitted to the unit for three weeks while her husband took a holiday. This sort of compassionate admission to the Hanbury Unit happened quite regularly, to give spouses a rest. Some patients love being allowed to dialyse in hospital as they don't have to set up and clean out the machine themselves.

Then there was a man suspected of drinking more than his fluid allowance and not dialysing regularly enough.

There is one patient on home dialysis who is Australian antigen positive. This means that he is a carrier of a virus that causes a lethal type of jaundice. If this infection got into the Hanbury Unit through his use of the machines it could develop into a killer epidemic. In the early days of dialysis units a number of hospitals were stricken with this disease and a number of staff as well as patients died of it. It is for fear of a carrier of this sort that the unit is completely sealed off from the outside world. It is a sterile area, and no one who has not had a blood test is allowed in. This patient complained that he could not sleep on the machine and so dialysed in the day.

One woman seemed to be getting anxious. She was not keeping to her diet. She had been admitted recently with a suspected pulmonary embolism from her fistula.

A middle-aged man was sinking into deeper and deeper depression, according to the social worker. 'I think he's a potential suicide,' the social worker said. The technician was brisk. 'He's just a big baby,' he said. 'He's no worse than he always was. He rings up all the time about some technical trouble or other. I've got to the point of fending him off.' A doctor suggested he should see a psychiatrist. 'At least he ought to be offered the opportunity.' Dr Goodwin said that a number of patients had problems with their sex lives. Some of the men had become impotent, at least temporarily, and many of the women said they had lost interest in sex.

The technicians in the dialysis unit are a crucial part of the team. As in other parts of the hospital, when treatments become more complex, and lives often depend as much on the absolute reliability of a machine as on the skill of a surgeon, the technician's status and importance is very great.

In the Hanbury Dialysis Unit the doctors work as a team with the nurses who train the patients, and the technicians, co-operating closely, asking each other's advice. Ultimate responsibility remains with the doctors, of course, but in the training of the patients to use the machines, and in the care of the patients once they are dialysing at home the nurses and technicians are almost as important.

Alan Hawkes is the chief renal technician. He attends most of the unit meetings about the dialysis patients, and he offers a quite different perspective on the cases. He is young, tough, dedicated, and a disciplinarian. His views provide a complete contrast to the soft generous approach of the social worker. He is treated by the doctors, nurses, and social workers as a sort of rough diamond, and his often harsh appraisal of the patients cuts through a lot of cotton wool in the thinking at these meetings.

He is in his early thirties, is studying for a BSc in electronics and was trained in radar. He then moved on to computers and started working on medical computers doing automatic blood analysis. It was while he was working on these that he heard that the new kidney dialysis unit was desperately in need of a technician.

'I thought I'd give it a try, and I stayed. We're always short-staffed here – run off our feet most of the time. It's very hard to get a renal technician. I'd say only about seventy-five per cent of the work is technical, and the rest is dealing with the patient and his problems. I can't take on a one hundred per cent technician. He has to be a psychologist too.

'It's almost a twenty-four hour a day job. You never leave it behind you. We're on call all day and three nights a week. Each of us has a book with all the patients in it, and we all know all of them very well.

'Every unit in every hospital is run differently. A renal technician has to be really qualified. After all, if he makes a mistake, it's a potential killer. Nothing man-made is perfect. We keep warning the patients of that. It's a complex machine, and it could be death if, say, an alarm doesn't work.

'Once a patient has been selected to go on to haemo-dialysis he is handed over to us in the unit to train. We judge a patient carefully as to what he can learn, how long it's going to take him to grasp, and how much we should tell him about the way the thing works. The dim ones we teach as little as possible. We tell them which is the front and back of the machine, and then just drill them with the routine parrot-fashion, over and over again. We're often surprised by the people who learn it fast, and those who we thought would do well are sometimes really hopeless.

'Once they go home we always expect a couple of months of continual panic phone calls. Usually you can deal with those on the phone – calm them down, and take them over the routine again. But if you go on getting those calls after the first few months, "nuisance calls" I call them, you start to ask yourself, is it the patient or the machine that's going wrong? And we get them back in here to watch them for a bit and sort things out. Of course we check them all every three months, and we analyse the dialysis fluid once a month.

'We have one or two troublesome patients who live a very long way away – takes ages to visit them, and when one of these acts up it's hard to keep your temper. Some of the patients feel special, and better than us. I tell them that anyone, a queen or a peasant can go on a machine. You have to stop and ask yourself why people are behaving like that. We have to anticipate them. I nearly hit a patient the other day who insisted I came out to look at his machine when I knew there was nothing the matter with it, and I was up to my neck in work. He had the nerve to say, "That's your job, to be on call to me."'

On the wall in Alan's office is a big chart with all the home dialysis patients marked on it. Every time they make a call or a complaint about their machine it is marked on the chart. 'We try to get ourselves some statistics,' he explained. 'We can see how well a patient is managing, or how well his machine is functioning by a glance at this chart. We mark beside each call whether it is a real malfunction or a patient's mistake.'

He ran his finger down the chart and pointed at a graph that showed peak times for calls. 'You'll notice that in very cold spells the machines start to act up. Cold affects them badly and we get a mass of calls. You can see other factors at work here too. Just before Christmas we get a deluge of calls. We work out a special Christmas timetable to get the patients to dialyse on the same nights to suit us and them best for getting in a good Christmas. The patients panic and think to themselves, "The technicians aren't going to be there. What will I do if my machine breaks down? I must get them in to mend that tiny fault I've been noticing for the last few months but haven't bothered about." The worst panic crisis came when an irresponsible newspaper published a report about a small strike going on at the hospital and said that the kidney technicians were coming out too. You should have heard the phone go!

'No, we're not unionized, none of the renal technicians in The London Hospital. Even contemplating it makes me shudder and go hot and cold at the thought of what would happen to the patients. You can't join a union if you would never in your life go on strike, if you wouldn't even threaten or pretend that you might strike. Lives would be endangered, the panic would be appalling and we are so short-staffed that we wouldn't have a hope of ever catching up with the work if we even stopped for a day.

'We're much better paid than we were. It was very bad when I started. Until two years ago a technician was only getting £1200, but last year we got a thirty-seven per cent rise, and this year it was thirty per cent. Technicians earn £3000 now. Mind you, I'd get at least another £2000 with my qualifications and expertise in private industry, but, I'm not interested in that now. For one thing, you can do research in private industry but you have to research into what they tell you. Here I am constantly trying out new things, ideas for improvements, and I'm free to work on what I want in that line.

'Of course this is a field where there's a lot of development work to be done, but you have to be careful what you say about it. The moment a report appears about the most hypo-thetical improvement to the machines, all the patients hear about it at once and they're on the phone demanding that they have whatever it is. But there is still the hope – and as a scientist I'll say the certainty – that we'll find better machines, and eventually it'll be easier and less painful. As long as the money for research keeps coming, there'll surely be a way.

'It's a lonely job a lot of the time. The lads have to work by themselves, and it can be a bit bleak for the technician out on the road all day. We have keys to all the patients' houses so we can get in and fix their machines while they're out or at work. You often don't see another living soul all day. We tell the patients to tie up their dogs when they go out, so we don't have any more nasty incidents with being attacked by the brutes.

'But you have plenty of excitement in this job too, a lot of drama. Nasty things go wrong with dialysis quite often, and my God, you have to dash to the scene when they do.

'Most of the police around this area recognize our little vans from this department, which is just as well. I'm not surprised. Only the other night I got a call from a patient, luckily not too far away, saying her husband's lines had come unfixed and there was a big leak and she couldn't fix it. You should have seen me go! I belted out and into the van, and I was away, doing ninety, I shouldn't wonder. The police came up behind me, flashing and the siren going, but I couldn't stop until they made me. I shouted at the policeman that I was off to help a kidney patient. I showed him my licence and documents and told him to lead the way and we'd discuss it later. Luckily he believed me, and he let me go, and led the way at a fair pace. When we got there I dashed up the stairs of the house and he came too. He took one look in the room, with blood everywhere, all over the floor and he nearly passed right out!'

Many of the kidney patients at The London never see a kidney machine or the dialysis unit.

There are four treatments for kidney failure – the kidney machine (or haemo-dialysis), peritoneal dialysis (a temporary and sometimes unpleasant method of washing out the blood by pumping a lot of fluid through a tube in the abdomen), kidney transplantation and 'conservative treatment'. Statistically, people on kidney machines live the longest, so this is usually considered to be the best treatment. People who have kidney transplants usually live a better life, but many patients may lose their transplants, or even their lives. A successful transplant may last for over ten years, but even when it fails the patient may still be able to return to dialysis or receive another transplant. Peritoneal dialysis at The London is always done in hospital and tends to lead to infections and complications; it is usually used for only a short time for those awaiting transplants, or a place in the dialysis unit.

Only those who are thought fit are offered the chance of haemo-dialysis. No patients are put on to kidney machines unless they can ultimately be sent home to dialyse themselves. Those waiting for transplants, but not thought suitable for home dialysis, are treated by peritoneal dialysis, which cannot be done indefinitely, and means the patient cannot afford to wait a long period for a well-matched kidney. The Hanbury Dialysis Unit is only used for training patients on the machines. This is because if other patients were put on to the machines they would use up the beds, perhaps for years, waiting for transplants, while many patients could have been trained and sent home in the time. Some patients are treated 'conservatively' and given none of these dramatic remedies.

The doctors have to make a harsh decision in the treatment they offer to their patients. Most of the patients don't realize the nature of the decision being made. They are told firmly, 'We think this is the right treatment for you,' and most assume that this decision has been reached on purely medical grounds.

In fact kidney machines, generally considered the best treatment, are usually offered only to people who are happily married, or have a close relative living with them. A patient on dialysis needs the help and support of a partner, and in the case of emergency, it is much safer to have someone there to call for help.

At The London Hospital few children are taken on for dialysis, though again, some hospitals do offer it. Dr Goodwin thinks the life too dreadful and cruel for very small children. Adolescents who can be helped by their parents may be offered dialysis, and often adapt remarkably well to it, though such compulsory overdependence on their parents at a time when they should be breaking away from them is deeply depressing and retarding for them emotionally. Married patients have to be settled and secure with their spouses before they are considered eligible. Dialysis puts an enormous strain on the best relationships. Then there is the consideration of general competence. 'You look at some of the patients, and you talk to them, and you know that they will just never learn to cope with it. Their lives are too disorganized and they could never adjust to such a rigorous routine. They would never learn to use the equipment in the first place. It requires enormous patience and discipline,' explained one doctor.

Some patients who are offered dialysis accept it, but come to regard it as a temporary measure and then ask for a transplant instead. They are told the chances of success and the chances of survival of transplant recipients, but they choose to take the risk of death in exchange for the chance of a happier life. The patients on haemo-dialysis are in the best position to get a good transplant if they want one. If it fails, and they survive, they can always go back on a kidney machine. Dialysis gives them the time to wait for a well-matched transplant – while those who are denied a machine are sometimes forced to accept whatever kidney comes along. Those who are not thought suitable for dialysis are simply told, 'A transplant would be the best thing for you.' The doctors know quite well that the chances of a perfectly matched kidney turning up in time are small.

Once a patient has been told he will get a transplant when a kidney becomes available, there is a choice. He can go on to the 'Category One' waiting list, or the 'Category Two' waiting list. On the 'Two' list he will only be offered a well-matched kidney, but he may have to wait a very long time for one. On the 'One' list he will be offered any compatible kidney, with a greater chance of rejection, but will be likely to get a kidney much sooner.

Patients already on a dialysis machine can afford to put themselves on the 'Two' list, while the rest are forced to go on to the 'One' list as they are in urgent need of a kidney.

So the privileged patients are those who are chosen to go on to a kidney machine either for ever, or while awaiting transplant.

After visiting the Hanbury Dialysis Unit and its patients, Dr Goodwin took me on his ordinary ward round in the main hospital, and I had a chance to ask Dr Brownjohn, his

Senior Registrar, what treatment he would give himself if his own kidneys failed. He drew a deep breath, 'I'd be a terrible patient,' he said and paused. 'If it was just me, I'd go for a transplant but as I have a family I'd be forced to choose dialysis as the life expectancy is longer, but I'd find it hard to bear.' We started in the Rothschild Ward.

In the first bed a man was lying still, semi-conscious, and the doctors stopped to read his notes near by. Dr Goodwin explained that the man had suffered a severe stroke and had advanced renal failure. 'He'll probably die in a few days,' he said. The ward Sister said he was very dehydrated. 'I don't think we should put a tube down him or put up a drip. It will only be a more unpleasant way to die,' he said. Someone asked if his wife knew he was going to die soon. 'Yes, but I don't think she's taken it in. She's not bright,' he said. 'She's suffering from the same disease and she's very frightened.'

The next patient was a West Indian, young and listless. He was lying on his bed propping up his head on one elbow. He was having peritoneal dialysis as he wasn't considered suitable for a machine.

'I'm afraid it can be a very unpleasant feeling, having your insides filled up with so much fluid,' Dr Goodwin said. The tube had become infected a few times. 'Well,' he said to the patient. 'We've decided to give you a transplant, haven't we?' The young man nodded gloomily. He looked almost indifferent, perhaps resentful. He didn't ask any questions or offer any remarks at all. 'I'm afraid it's just a question now of waiting until one turns up. Do you understand that?' He nodded again slightly and gave a small shrug, as if it didn't matter much to him one way or the other. 'I know you want to go home,' Dr Goodwin persisted, 'but you're really not well enough yet.' The group moved away from his bed.

'The trouble with a lot of these patients is that they have great trouble in understanding and accepting that they are ill. Kidney failure often happens suddenly to people who have apparently been quite healthy, until they collapse one day. It takes a long time for them to believe that they really are ill.

That young man just wants to go home and get out of here. He doesn't believe it. He thinks that the peritoneal dialysis is unnecessary, and that we are inflicting it on him for no reason. He thinks everything would be all right if we left him alone.'

How long, I asked, would he have to wait for his transplant?

'Possibly a year, for even a bad match,' Dr Goodwin said. Would he last that long? 'Hopefully he will, but peritoneal dialysis is sometimes difficult to continue for so long, and he may not survive until a transplant comes along.'

Why couldn't he have a kidney machine? 'I don't think he could cope with one. It would be cruel to even try it, because it wouldn't work, and we'd regret ever having started.' In fact, a year later this patient was still receiving peritoneal dialysis in the ward, although he was spending most of his time at home. No transplant had become available yet, but he was doing well and had learned to accept the situation.

In the next bed was a man in his mid sixties lying quietly with a greyish-yellow face and white cracked lips. He was suffering from partial renal failure. Like a lot of renal patients, his initial complaint had been something different, but the course of his illness had damaged his kidneys. 'He had an aortic aneurysm. They took him into the operating theatre to repair it, but just as they opened him up, it exploded and splattered blood all over everywhere. He almost died. For thirty-five minutes they cut off the supply of blood to his kidneys, severely damaging them. He'll probably just about get by with the little function there is left in them.'

Dr Goodwin said that in many of the patients referred to him by other departments of the hospital, their kidney disease was a complication of some other condition, or its treatment.

In the next bed was a small anxious-looking man. 'We thought he would be suitable for dialysis but the more we see of him and his wife, the more we doubt it. They are both very nervous. Whenever I talk to her about her husband's illness all she can tell me about is herself, and how she's already on so much valium. She's only interested in her own neurosis and I can't get in a word about her husband.' He paused for a moment.

'Many people tell us that we shouldn't make this sort of decision. But if you put someone on to dialysis and you get it all set up, and then they can't cope, the treatment can be worse than the disease.'

In the next ward was a woman who was training for haemodialysis. She was going to have a machine installed at home once she had learned to use it. First she had already been given a transplant which had failed and had to be removed after a week. She had had her own kidneys removed and patients without their kidneys do less well than those who keep them. They tend to be more anaemic. She held out her arm for Dr Goodwin to look at. It had been operated on to make a fistula to increase the flow of blood to make needling easier for using the machine.

In the next bed was a fat woman in a short green nylon frilly nightie. She was middle-aged, and had bitten her nails down to the quick. She was waiting for a transplant. 'Are there any questions you would like to ask?' Dr Goodwin asked.

'Well, yes,' she said, looking down at the bed covers. 'If I get a kidney, and it "takes", how long will it last?'

Dr Goodwin patted her arm. 'Don't worry,' he said. 'It'll last the rest of your life.'

Last the rest of her life? True enough, but how long?

Neither Dr Goodwin nor the woman noticed the nonsense of what he had just said, luckily. She smiled and was reassured. People on the edge of death tend to be mercifully uninquiring.

'It always amazes me how little they ask. It has nothing to do with education or social background, but people hardly ever ask a question as bold as that woman's. I suppose they don't want to know.'

In a small room behind a large glass window that gave on to the corridor of one of the big kidney wards lay a girl in her late twenties, Alison. She was a pretty girl with a slightly puffy face – a classic feature of transplanted patients. She smiled at the doctors who went by her room. Outside in the corridor was a telephone for people who were passing to talk to her, without having to wash and put on gowns, for the room itself was a sterile area. She had had a kidney transplant a month before, and was still on the immunity-suppressing drugs that make patients so vulnerable. The most common cause of death in kidney transplant recipients is overwhelming infection.

Standing in the corridor looking through the glass, like at an animal in the zoo, Dr Goodwin told me about her.

At fifteen Alison had developed acute nephritis which began as a sore throat which then affected her kidneys, a complaint which particularly affects young people. Dr Goodwin was then a houseman and he had been her doctor for the fourteen years since then, and knew her well. She hadn't been an easy patient, perhaps because she became so ill in the middle of adolescence. She was a middle-class girl from the Home Counties, and was often critical of the treatment she was getting at the hospital. The last year had been a terrible time for her.

I went into the room in mask, cap and gown and she smiled and turned the sound off the television set she was watching.

'It's a funny thing – sick in a way. They've been having a kidney transplant drama on *General Hospital* all this week. Of course they get it all wrong. I know most of the technical things and they skate over it all.' She put down her knitting, and slowly pulled herself up on her pillows.

She had a vague and slightly apathetic air – I wasn't sure if that was part of her illness, or her usual personality. She began to talk about her life.

Ever since her first illness at fifteen her kidneys had been badly damaged. 'I had stopped coming to the hospital for a long time, as I was sure I was getting better. I stopped believing that there was anything much the matter with me. I used to come regularly to have blood levels checked, and they did find I had a high urea level [a substance that builds up in the body if kidneys are not functioning well, or if a patient with impaired kidneys doesn't keep to the prescribed diet]. I got casual about the diet. I hate the protein-free bread – crumbly and sticky. I think my diet really went wrong over Christmas, and I was cooking a lot for my boy-friend. When you cook you taste things, and you don't count the tastes in your allowance for the day. It just gradually built up and then suddenly I became very ill, for the first time since I was fifteen, just after I came back from a holiday. I had an overload of salt and my heart was going mad. They gave me diuretics to bring down my blood pressure. They wired me up to a monitor and I could see my heart going crazy and I was scared. Strange doctors I didn't know kept coming and listening to different parts of me, not just the kidney doctors whom I knew well. Then all these students kept crowding in to have a listen and I couldn't bear it. I listened to everything I could that they were saying, or whispering about me. I couldn't make sense of most of it, but you know how you twist things you don't understand? I imagined everything and anything and I was terrified. I don't think they knew how much they were frightening me. I asked questions and didn't understand the answers properly, but thought I did, and imagined the worst. For instance someone said something about systolic and I thought they were talking about a cyst, and that was a euphemism for cancer. I kept mishearing.

'Then the day came, I'll never forget it, it was a Friday. Dr Marsh came in and he sat on the bed and he said, "We've got to do something about you. We've got to give you a new kidney." I went numb for a week.

'I had always known my kidneys weren't good but I didn't think anything would really happen about them until well into middle age. There was no way I thought anything would happen to me now, while I'm young and strong. Not to me.

'No, there was never any choice or question about the sort of treatment I'd get. They never really discussed the chance that I might go on to a kidney machine. They just said that the best thing for me would be a kidney transplant. They said as I was unmarried, living alone in a flat, and as I liked travelling a lot and I'm used to being quite free and easy, a new kidney would be best for me, which seems reasonable, I think. But I was scared nearly out of my mind. I'd never had an operation of any kind until then and I thought I'd die as soon as I went under an anaesthetic. Dr Goodwin just smiled and said I could die just as easily crossing the road, which is true if you think about it like that.

'They told me I'd have to have a small operation to put a peritoneal dialysis tube into my stomach. But the thought of being cut open was almost too much for me. Some people don't mind much, but I do, just the thought of it. Another thing, being in a teaching hospital scares me too. I'm always afraid of getting a surgeon who hasn't done it before. Same with the nurses – if one comes in who I don't know to give me an injection or take out some stitches I always say straight away, right out, "Have you ever done it before?" and if they said no I'd send them away. I don't want them learning on me.' She looked petulant as she shifted her pillows into a better position.

'Peritoneal dialysis is awful. You have a nasty tube that sticks right out of your stomach. It keeps blocking up all the time and getting infected. You have to come up to the hospital three times a week to be dialysed. I just lie back and shut my eyes. They give you a local anaesthetic and you just feel a sort of pummelling of the hands when they do it, then the weight of all those pints of water flushing in and out of you. I keep my eyes shut but I don't have to use much imagination to know what's going on.'

I didn't, of course, ask her whether it had ever occurred to her that this suffering on peritoneal dialysis was quite unnecessary. She could have come into the hospital three times a week and had haemo-dialysis instead, which, though no treat, is more comfortable. But because of the hospital's policy of never letting the haemo-dialysis machines be used by those who do not qualify to train to have the machines at home, all those who are not on home dialysis but who are awaiting kidney transplants must go through the inconvenience and discomfort of having a tube in their stomach all the time.

However Alison was lucky. It was not long before a kidney was offered to her.

'I got a phone call at one o'clock. I'd been feeling really ill for a long time, and when the call came it was such a shock.

There again you just go numb when someone rings you in the middle of the night and tells you to rush round for a major operation. I started feeling sick. My boy-friend took me round to the hospital and I had all the blood tests, and I was scrubbed and shaved, and then they gave me a pre-med, but they kept warning, "You may wake up and find nothing's been done, if the kidney isn't OK." I remember going into the theatre. I didn't want to see anything. I didn't want to see anything nasty, or any machinery or any surgeons. I did open my eyes and saw this young doctor, and I asked if he'd done one before, and if he was too tired at this time of night to do a good job? Then I was asleep. I knew the kidney was coming from Hammersmith, but that was all.

'Well, I didn't keep that kidney for long. You can tell if it starts to function by your urine output, and they never tried to tell me it was working. I got a blood clot in the vein leading to the new kidney, and it turned out that no blood was getting through at all and the kidney went septic.

'They took it out a few days later. I was in hospital a month and the time was slow passing. Everything seemed to go wrong. I noticed then that these steroids they give you change your character completely. I'm different now. I used to be very outspoken. I'd run everything down. Everything round me had to be perfect. But steroids make you passive. I do knitting and tapestry now, which I'd never have had the patience for before.'

When she came out of hospital after the unsuccessful transplant she went back to live with her parents, commuted to London to work, and spent three nights a week being given peritoneal dialysis. But everything went badly and she kept getting infections and the tube kept blocking. 'Then they put in this flexible one which was a bit better as at least it lies flat against you when not in use, and doesn't stick out,' she said.

Then she became very ill, and was rushed to hospital with peritonitis, from the tube. She must have been reaching the end of the road when the chance of a second kidney came up, shortly after she had gone home.

'A voice on the telephone at one-thirty in the morning said, "May I speak to Alison Weston," and I knew what it was right away. Dr Goodwin just said to me, "Hello Alison, we've got a kidney for you. Get here as soon as possible." I said I'd take a taxi, and I grabbed a nightdress and toothbrush and ran.

'And this time was different. I told myself it had to be. With the first kidney transplant, I refused any painkillers at all or any sedatives as I thought somehow in the back of my mind that they might affect the transplant and make it less likely to work. I was in terrible pain all the time it was going septic, but I wouldn't take anything.

'But this time, the second time, I wasn't half so hopeful, so I just took whatever I could, and anyway, I've hardly had any pain at all. I was in a trance at first, and then I just decided to make my day in here into a routine, doing knitting, sewing, reading and watching television for an exact time every day, to take my mind off thinking about it.'

She paused and gazed at the silent television where now a male singer was crooning silently into a microphone showing all his clean white teeth in close up.

'I have made one mistake this time. I asked who was next door, and they told me it was a man who had been given another kidney. I asked how his was doing and it seems his started to work right away, straight off like that. Mine is slow and sluggish and that depresses me. I've had to have more peritoneal dialysis but it hasn't been too painful. But now it really looks as if I won't need any more as the kidney is beginning to work. It's good news, although they can't be completely sure for about five weeks or so.

'But that's always been my trouble with this hospital, I ask too many questions and frighten myself with the answers. It's better not to know anything at all, and to shut your ears to whispers, rumours and gossip. That was the trouble when I was in the big open ward. You'd sit at the table and ask people what they were in for, and maybe they'd have the same thing as you and they'd tell you frightening things you don't want to know.'

It happened by chance that Dr Goodwin, a couple of nurses and some medical students were passing by Alison's glass window on the way out of the ward at the end of a round. They paused to look through at us, to wave and smile. Then in a huddle they stopped to talk.

'What's she telling her?' I heard Dr Goodwin say.

'Goodness only knows, she's been in there long enough,' another doctor said.

'She wasn't the absolutely perfect patient to pick to talk to a journalist,' the Sister said. Alison laughed, and I laughed too.

'That's my little secret,' said Alison. 'They all think this room is soundproof, but I can hear every word they say. They don't realize because it doesn't seem to work the other way round. They can't hear me. But I always hear everything they're saying when they stand out there and discuss my case. Shall I tell them now? I think I will.' She picked up her telephone beside the bed, and Dr Goodwin picked up his on the other side of the glass. 'I've always been able to hear every word you say!' she said. And he was suitably taken aback. Later when he asked, I told him that it was true, and he felt uncomfortable.

Alison went on with her story. 'Of course one of the things that probably did me a lot of harm before my kidneys got really bad, was when I went to a new doctor. I needed a National Health one in London – as the family doctor who knew me was private and practised near where my parents live. This new doctor was told that I was a kidney patient. I went to him with a cold and he prescribed tetracycline three times a day. It turns out that this drug is very bad indeed for kidney patients, and it did me harm. The doctor should have known that, but he didn't.'

She was staring at the television again. 'I'm determined not to be too optimistic but this time it really looks as if everything may be all right. How lovely to be free of this place!'

Alison didn't talk about life expectancy. Dr Goodwin said that she, like most other patients, had never asked. 'The facts are these,' he said. 'After five years fifty per cent of the transplant patients are still alive, while seventy per cent of the haemo-dialysis patients have survived.'

A few weeks later Alison died of complications following the rejection of her kidney.

There was a meeting that day to discuss the transplant patients. In the absence of Dr Goodwin, Dr Brownjohn was presiding. The first case was that of a sixteen-year-old girl who spoke no English.

'She is very ill again, and I'm afraid she'll have to go back on peritoneal dialysis,' Dr Brownjohn said. 'But I hate to do it to her.'

'Last time she cried and cried,' Ros Levenson said.

'She's been very unlucky and has had so many infections with it. She's had a very bad time indeed,' Dr Brownjohn said.

Ros said, 'None of her family speak a word of English, and I don't think they understand at all what's going on.'

'Certainly we must consider that the quality of her life is not good,' Dr Brownjohn said carefully.

There was a moment's silence in the room before Ros said, 'But we must realize too that she looks at her life from a different point of view. From what I see of them I think they are a loving protective family, and that somehow, despite everything, even despite her dreadful illness, she is happy. But she is miserably isolated in hospital. She doesn't understand anything and she cries a lot of the time.'

More for my benefit than anyone else's, as everyone there knew the patient well already, Dr Brownjohn said, 'We've already absolutely had to rule out a kidney machine. That family couldn't even begin to manage. So now we have to look at this thing straight in the eye. Are we causing more suffering than anything else? We are doing no good to that girl or her family at the moment. Of course we hope and hope that a transplant will come up. That would be the only satisfactory answer – but what are we to do?' He paused. 'We could decide to do nothing. To wait and hope for a transplant, and to do nothing in the meantime, on the grounds that her suffering is too great. As far as peritoneal dialysis is concerned, I think we are inflicting an unnecessary torture. The death of a sixteen-year-old girl in that family is a dreadful tragedy, but she is not a mother or a breadwinner, with people depending on her. For her own sake, should we go on dialysing?'

Ros Levenson said again, 'I think she is happy. . . . But I agree that I wouldn't like to see her back on peritoneal dialysis.'

'Are we agreed to do nothing more, until a transplant?' Dr Brownjohn asked. It seemed almost certain that they would decide to stop treating the girl – that is, to let her die in peace unless a transplant came in time, rather than to force her through more suffering and have her probably die anyway – but a decision was not finally taken at this meeting.

No one in the hospital wanted to talk about death. For most of the staff it means only failure – they are preoccupied with keeping bodies alive. The only person I met who discussed it at length was Carol, another social worker from the neuro-surgery department. The social workers are employed to worry about people as people, not as bodies.

Carol, echoed what most of the social workers say. 'It would be arrogant to think you can really do much good. All I am is a sounding board. People can formulate their thoughts by talking to me when perhaps they can't talk to anyone else. The doctors are in a hurry, the nurses are busy, but they know we are there just to talk. We arrive at the crisis point in some-one's life. Their problem is often something they can't talk about to their family. Perhaps a strong young man, active breadwinner, has an accident, and overnight is turned into a wheelchair cripple. He may want to talk about his family and his relationships, and to think out how his role has changed. He may want to ask questions he doesn't dare ask the doctor, and I can go and ask for him. For instance about sex. I know that man is going through the most terrible time, and I have to remember that nothing I do will radically alter his position. It's just that if a patient can resolve some of the things in his mind at a time of crisis, you may save him from much greater mental anguish later. Perhaps the thought that you can't do much harm either makes the job possible and bearable. You can't shoulder someone else's burdens, and it is arrogant to imagine you can.'

Carol describes an important part of her work as being an intermediary. She is a befriender acting as go-between for the patient and the institution. She is not in uniform, and does not belong to the 'them' that patients often identify as a threatening force.

Nurses sometimes need protecting from the patients. 'Quite often it happens that a patient who discovers he is dying, or has become crippled is full of anger. Someone who has had a brain tumour removed and has become partially paralysed may well blame everyone around him. He will be full of hostility and violence. This sort of violence is very hard for the nurses to cope with, particularly the young eighteen- and nineteen-year-olds. Sometimes the patient becomes unpopular in the ward; you have to explain it to the nurses, if you can. Mostly they're very understanding. It's easy for us, as we go in and out of the wards and may only see a patient twice a day, but the nurses have to cope with the awfulness of his terrible situation and his impossible behaviour all the time. They have to have defences. Some of the young ones can feel very threatened by the sight of a young person stricken with an incurable illness, and will put up strong defences to protect themselves against a patient. We have to be intermediaries.'

Trying to soften up the doctors and nurses is her hardest job, she says. 'Some of the nurses have strong religious faith, and they manage best. They aren't afraid themselves, and don't feel threatened. They are nice and have plenty of defences which are not directed against the patient. Some of the others say they just don't think about it. Perhaps some of the unimaginative ones don't, but I think they all do at some time or other. I don't know how they cope with all that suffering all day long without cutting themselves off. "Why is Mrs X making such a fuss when she's nothing like as ill as Mrs Y?" a nurse may grumble. You have to point out that people are different, and that anyway, Mrs X is still a very ill woman, and the fact there's someone more ill next door doesn't affect her own feelings very much.'

She stopped to think about the nurses.

'We often think we should try and educate some of the surgeons. They can be the worst,' she said. 'I have to really fight sometimes in trying to explain why a patient isn't ready to go home even though his scar may be healed enough medically. But then, I have to stop and remind myself of what the surgeons are doing. How much could they really take if they didn't detach themselves from the patients? Wouldn't they crack up altogether? Isn't it like trying to get a butcher to join the RSPCA and carry on with his work all the same? They get a lot of abuse from the patients too – patients feel the surgeon has maimed them, after an amputation.'

The social worker may find herself being an intermediary with the patient's family too. The family may be horrified and unable to cope. She can listen to their worst horrors and fears and guilt. She can talk them into discussing the future, what they will do, how they will manage, into visualizing realistically what the future will be like. She often gets to know the relatives of those about to die and visits them at home after the death.

The social worker will, too, be making an assessment of the family, deciding whether they can manage the patient at home. If she thinks the family cannot take on a wheelchair case then she will have to try to find a bed in a home for the chronic sick, or possibly a home for the terminally ill.

'It is extremely difficult to find beds anywhere for the young [under fifty] chronically sick. If you have a person who will have to be nursed for the rest of her life, and she is, perhaps only in her thirties, you have to find a home that will agree to have one of its beds permanently blocked for perhaps the next forty years. This is where the greatest shortage is in the National Health. They built thousands of maternity beds in the last decade, and all sorts of other hospitals, but care of the chronic sick has been left almost exclusively to the voluntary organizations like the Cheshire Homes.'

The waiting list for places like the Cheshire Homes is long. It usually takes a year, Carol reckons, for her to get a patient into one. It costs the local authority £67 a week to send a patient there. It costs the National Health £300 a week to keep him in an acute bed at The London Hospital. Carol has several patients under her care who have been waiting months and months, the consultants desperate to vacate their beds, and the patients needing no further special care. The patients suffer in a general ward where there are no special facilities and everyone is coming and going all the time. As so often, the spending of a little money to make more chronic beds would save a great deal in the proper use of acute beds. Recently Carol had a brain-damaged young man in the ward, requiring no treatment, and he stayed for over a year, as no bed could be found for him.

St Joseph's Hospice which used to be called 'for incurables' and is still remembered as such by the local community, will take a number of long-stay patients, but mostly it is for those about to die. It is run independently by Catholic nuns. They do not like to take a patient unless the doctors are reasonably sure that he will die within the next three months. 'Although it sounds a grim place to send anyone, in fact it isn't. Not *everyone* there is going to die, as they do mix in a few long-stay patients with the terminally ill,' Carol explained. 'I have to do a lot of persuading, though. It's hard to get patients and their relatives to accept the idea of going there. Of course if they won't accept it no one's going to force them. Usually what persuades them is when I tell them about the very highly specialized treatment for pain relief available at St Joseph's. No one is cured there, but nearly all of them are greatly relieved of pain.

'In this hospital all the emphasis goes on curing. If someone is in pain they may give them large doses of drugs that dope them up a lot. The patients usually have to keep asking for it, and the nurses are busy. They only get it given when the pain has come back. At St Joseph's all the doctors' energies are used on finding the right delicate balance of drugs to keep a patient out of pain, but not more doped than he wants to be. The patients with terminal cancer who are in great pain sometimes have cordotomies done by the neuro-surgeons here before they go to St Joseph's. This is an operation in the spine to numb and ease the pain in some parts of the body. This operation does cause some trouble: the pain stops suddenly, and excruciating pain is, mercifully, rather quickly forgotten once it is over. The patient is left perhaps unable to use one arm very well, or slightly paralysed in some part of the body. Then he will blame the hospital and resent the surgeons for what they have done, forgetting that he begged for anything that would relieve the pain. That is a difficult situation for us to deal with.'

Carol is a young girl, like most of the social workers, and has worked at the hospital for two and a half years. She has a degree but is not a trained social worker. She is gentle and perceptive.

'You face people dying all the time. It doesn't make it any more acceptable. It doesn't make the thought of my own death any more bearable. Of course you can't identify with them. You just try to follow what's going on in their minds, and be sensitive to their mood of the moment. Most people with cancer half-know what's going to happen, but then they also don't know. One day a patient will say something a little oblique, but which recognizes her approaching death. One woman the other day suddenly said to me how sad she was that although she had been so happily married, she had no children; there would be nothing left of her by which her husband would remember her. I listened, and we talked about it a bit. When I went to see her later that day, she was talking to me about all the energetic gardening she was going to do as soon as she got home and was better.' She paused a moment to think about it.

'It may sound odd to you, but sometimes there are marvellous moments. There is a patient in the ward at the moment who is dying of cancer. She has been suffering excruciating pain for years and years now. She had stopped being a person. No one around her seemed to remember any more what she was once like. She had been quite overwhelmed by the pain in the whole of her upper half, and there was nothing left of her but her suffering. She has just had a cordotomy, which has quite suddenly lifted the pain away from her. The suffering she has lived under all these years has fallen away, and she is almost afraid. She doesn't know any longer what she is. I sit and talk with her and each day I can see her trying to struggle back into a personality, trying to find herself, to remember what she was before. It is a very difficult re-adjustment, but it really is marvellous to see a whole new person emerge, slowly and tentatively flowering into a real human being again.

'Sometimes patients who have undergone great physical and mental change like to bring out photographs of themselves before their illness – they are saying to me, "Look I'm a person – just like you – this is what I *really* look like."'

Social workers attend psychological lectures on subjects which are relevant to their work. 'The other day a man was explaining to us how in fact none of us can conceive of our own death. The subconscious refuses to accept and cannot accept the concept of its own annihilation. I don't think I can. Perhaps these patients don't either. It's hard to tell. Sometimes someone says to me, "I don't seem to be getting much better," and I know they are dying. I try not to give false assurances. I say something like, "Well, what do you feel about that?" You try to get them to talk. At least they aren't expecting anything of you. You are not a doctor and you aren't going to make them better. They put you into whatever role they see you in that day.'

One of the problems she encounters is that doctors do not always tell patients what is the matter with them. 'I'm afraid this isn't done on a personal assessment basis. Usually it is a matter of policy with some doctors and not with others. It's very arbitrary and depends on the doctor's attitude more than the patient's state of mind.'

Some patients can't cope at all with the knowledge. 'One woman I am visiting at home at the moment, who comes in and out of the ward at regular intervals, is very young, with a small daughter. Quite often she flings herself at me and screams, "You won't let me die, will you? I can't die! I won't die, it can't happen to me, not ME." I find that appalling. I think I might behave like that myself. I don't know what to do about it. I sit with her and try and calm her down. But then some days she tells me that she's better, that the cancer has gone; she knows really that it's still there. I do think all this is worse for the doctors. That woman knows I can't cure her, but she probably thinks the doctors can, or could, or should, or might if they tried a bit harder. It's far worse for them to face someone like that. Perhaps that's why a lot of them don't stop to talk to patients for long. It's scary if it's your own responsibility. I want these patients to feel it's all right to burst out and say they can't bear it and it's all right too, to be unbearable.'

Theories about dying, and coping with death is left mainly to the social workers. I couldn't find a doctor who would discuss it in any depth – even in the kidney department where many people were dying.

The kidney transplant side of the nephrology department's work is the most exciting and sometimes the most rewarding, but given how many people die in hospital it is rather a surprising and disturbing fact that so few kidneys become available for transplantation. Doctors tend to think obsessively about their own corner of medicine, their own patients and forget about what goes on elsewhere. In the main it is doctors who can be blamed for the lack of kidneys offered to those needing transplants.

When a kidney is made available anywhere in the country its details are relayed at once to a special computer in Bristol. On that computer are all the names of the people all over the country who are waiting for a transplant, and beside their names it is stated which Category they are. If there is anyone on the Category Two list for whom the kidney is a perfect match, then he will get first chance. If there is no one who exactly matches, then it will be offered to any compatible match on the Category One list. The hospital that provides the kidneys still has the option to keep one, or sometimes both of them for its own patients, although in doing so the patient receiving it may get a poor match and a patient elsewhere for whom it would have been a good match has to go without.

Dr Brownjohn explained the system. 'A call will come through that there is a potential kidney for one of our patients. It will be transported to us either by public transport, Securicor or by volunteers with their own small aeroplanes through the St John Ambulance organization within twelve hours. It is perfused with a chemical solution and put on ice so that it doesn't require so much oxygen. If it is left for too long, damage starts to be done to it. Nearly all transplants arrive with us at night.

'Most kidneys come from patients who have been on respirators, usually with brain damage. Occasionally we get kidneys from our own Intensive Therapy Unit, but not often.

'There is a problem now about harvesting kidneys. People are living longer now and the kidneys of elderly people are unsuitable for transplantation. Many of the younger people who die who would have been suitable donors develop kidney damage during their terminal illness.

'In the last year only four kidneys have been made available to us from this hospital. We find it very difficult to solicit for kidneys. We did have a very keen young transplant surgeon here not long ago, and he made a tremendous effort to get other departments in the hospital to realize how desperately we need kidneys. It's a difficult thing to do, and the doctors thought he was a bit of a vampire, I think. Anyway, his campaign fell flat, and we still aren't getting the kidneys we should.

'It isn't difficult to get relatives of someone who has just died to agree. They almost always say yes, when we explain how the kidneys could give life to two people. Death takes people in different ways. Sometimes they jump at you and kick and scratch. Once the transplant has been done, we get few inquiries from the relatives of the donor.'

All patients waiting for a transplant have a telephone, in

case the call should come.

'As soon as news comes through that there is a kidney for someone, we call the patient and tell him to rush round here as soon as possible,' Dr Brownjohn said. 'We get him completely ready for the operation before the kidney arrives. It is vital not to lose a moment. We have to take a blood test and ensure that the patient has no cold or flu, as that would endanger his life when he is later given heavy doses of immuno-suppressive drugs and will have no resistance to the smallest infection. Then we have to wait right up to the last minute for the kidney to arrive.

'We even get the patient into the anaesthetic room after a pre-med sometimes before we decide what state the kidney is in, and whether we can go ahead.'

The doctors in the nephrology department then hand their patient over to the transplant surgeons. They will play little part in the operation itself, though normally one of them will be present. After the operation the patient is cared for by both the physicians and the surgeons who did the operation.

Afterwards it may soon become apparent that the kidney is being rejected, and if anti-rejection treatment is unsuccessful, it may be removed quickly. It may take up to six weeks before the doctors know whether the kidney will function successfully.

As kidneys are so scarce, I asked whether patients' relatives ever volunteered one of their own live kidneys. For those who are on kidney machines and are awaiting transplants, the delay is tolerable, but for the others who have been denied machines and who will die if a transplant doesn't come soon, the waiting must be agonizing for all around them.

'No, oddly enough it doesn't often occur to relatives to offer a kidney of their own. I don't know why not,' Dr Brownjohn said. 'Of course a kidney from a live donor would have a vastly improved chance of doing well. We would get the donor into the theatre with the recipient and the time the kidney was out of the body would be minimal. There is always the risk to the donor, but the best-matched live-donor kidneys do very well indeed.'

It happened that during that week The London Hospital illustrated newsletter featured a huge front-page article about a patient who had had a successful transplant. She was photographed beaming and gaily told the readers how her life had been transformed. It was an article that made many people in the hospital wince. The newsletter had just been handed over to a public relations firm to edit and the story smacked of the worst kind of 'miracles of modern medicine' mythology. But there is little doubt that when transplants work they are a dynamic and satisfying form of treatment.

It is a dangerous treatment, but when the alternative is a kidney machine, there is something to be said for that. If it works it is a once-only treatment, worth spending a lot of money and energy on, because the patient will be well again, without the need for a stringent diet, or dialysis. He will live an absolutely normal life, at least for a while. This is not one of those dramatic expensive treatments that leave people alive but still very ill and which force us to ask if the treatment is worse than the disease, and if we are getting our medical priorities right.

The sad thing about kidney transplants is that so few of them can be carried out while doctors fail to take seriously the need to obtain donor kidneys. If as many kidneys were offered as are available the chance of each operation being successful would be much greater: the matches would be likely to be better. It is hard to understand why hundreds of kidneys aren't on offer every day to the Bristol kidney computer. The only explanation is that doctors can rarely be bothered about hypothetical patients, people not actually in their care. The life of some dying, but distant, kidney-disease sufferer seems not to impinge on their consciences. The relatively minor embarrassment of having to ask bereaved relatives for permission is enough to stop them from bothering about lives they could easily save.

There is, at the time of writing, some hope that the law might be changed, and permission of relatives might not be needed in order to remove parts of the body from someone who has just died. (I feel I own my body, and when I die I see no reason why I should suddenly belong to my next of kin.) The kidney donor cards that more and more people are beginning to carry around with them have no legal validity, and doctors cannot remove kidneys from someone carrying one, without a relative's permission.

They are being used and distributed more as a public relations exercise to demonstrate the sort of support there would be for a change in the law. But in fact, the doctors alone could easily procure enough kidneys from their patients who die in hospital.

8

Old Age

Most of us are born and most of us die in hospital. It is our temple of life and death. But it is a bad place to spend the last days. That is not what it is there for. The geriatric department at The London struggles hard to keep people out for as long as possible.

The Catholic Church has a prayer for 'The Happy Death' – and I would add to that a line or two about not dying in hospital in a geriatric ward. I was glad that the only death I was aware of while I visited that department was of an old woman who had never been in hospital before.

Her name was Violet Blanche Miller. She was brought in one bright morning to the Mercer Ward at the Mile End Hospital, a separate hospital which became part of The London in 1968. She was wheeled into a single room at one side of the ward, unconscious. At first they weren't even sure of her name. The milkman had raised the alarm when the previous day's milk was found still standing on the pavement. The police broke into her flat and found her alone, unconscious on the floor.

She was a round handsome woman, probably in her late seventies. Her firm round cheeks had a rosiness even while she was unconscious. She seemed peaceful, even happy, with what looked like half a smile on her face. She was like everyone's favourite granny. The smile, which never wore off, wasn't I think so much of a smile, as a happy expression. She looked like a contented person, whose wrinkles came from smiles not frowns.

While I watched her being put into the bed I hoped and

hoped that she would soon spring to life. I felt I would have liked her. The nurses liked her too. One of them stroked her face, and brushed some strands of grey hair from her eyes. They called her from time to time, but got no response at all.

She lay in the bed on her side, looking quite naturally asleep, and only lightly asleep. Patients going into the operating theatre look much deader than she. I was optimistic.

No one knew how long she had been lying on the floor. I was shocked when at first they diagnosed her as having taken a massive overdose of anti-depressants. That didn't fit my picture of her.

'We all have strong ideas of what a person is like when they are unconscious,' said a nurse. 'If you like the look of one, the chances are that they turn out to be a bit of a disappointment. While you're hoping they'll come out of it you really involve yourself and imagine someone nice.'

When the woman was identified, and her son was interviewed, the doctors found out a little more about her. She had never been in hospital before, and had not been ill. They got the impression that he hardly ever visited her – perhaps once a fortnight at the most. They could find out little about her social life and friends – but they did discover she took anti-depressants, perhaps because she was lonely.

She just lay there for several days, her teeth in a plastic mug on the sink of the little room. She had no other personal possessions with her.

The geriatric department is sprawled across the borough, housed in four small hospitals. The London does not allocate a single geriatric bed to their main hospital. However there has been discussion about changing this for some time. The department's headquarters at the Mile End Hospital are bright and pleasant, but the other three parts, at Bethnal Green Hospital, St Clement's and St Matthew's are grim. St Matthew's is the worst. It is a slightly renovated work-house used mainly for long-stay patients. St Clement's is a mental hospital with a number of psycho-geriatric beds mainly for the severely demented aged.

One of the reasons geriatrics get such short shrift in a big teaching hospital is that it isn't a real academic speciality. The only definition the Department of Health can produce for a geriatric is 'one who is under the care of a geriatrician'. Some doctors do not recognize geriatrics as a separate discipline but regard it as a bureaucratic invention of the NHS. Since fifty per cent of people in hospital are over the age of sixty-five, age alone does not necessarily identify the geriatric patient. Old age is not a disease, but an accumulation of complaints, any one of which could be treated by a consultant in another field.

Dr Silver is the consultant geriatrician. He is a quiet, mild and serious man, dedicated, and with little personal ambition. His job is quite different to that of any other consultant in the hospital. It is not so much consultant, as social worker. He is head of the Tower Hamlets Geriatric Service. While most doctors at the hospital, if they choose, can put their patients into an imaginary bag and make a small hole to inspect just the leg or arm, or lung that interests them, most of Dr Silver's time is spent in assessing what his patients can do, where and how they should live. Actual treatment is only part of his work. It is the only department in the hospital to be entirely based on the local community. No geriatrics ever get referred to this department from outside the borough. There are no interesting and complicated cases to be forwarded to this part of the hospital from all over the country, as in many other departments.

Over the years Dr Silver gets to know most of his patients well. They come back, with greater and greater frequency, each time a little worse than before, each time with a few more complaints. His out-patients' clinic is possibly even more important than his work in the wards. He is scrutinizing his patients carefully, checking to see that they are still fit enough to survive on their own, and sometimes, with great reluctance, deciding to admit them.

Bethnal Green Hospital is a dingy place. Attempts have been made to make it look better – surprising bright yellow walls or modern doors try to disguise the dreariness.

There was already a small queue of people outside the door as Dr Silver arrived for the first out-patient appointment of the day.

His room was small with a fuzzy glass window set a little too high in the wall. There were big pipes up one side. It looked exactly like a prison cell. There were two small rooms leading off it each with a bed in them.

Many of Dr Silver's patients had mixed and not very specific complaints. He would watch them, each time they came back, get to know some of them quite well, and perhaps, as each visit they got a little worse, and a little less able to cope, take them into hospital and, in the end, see them die.

When he had sat down and glanced at the names on the files on his desk he told the Sister to send in the first patient.

First came a new patient, wheeled in a hospital wheel-chair by her daughter. Mrs Brown was wearing a nightdress, slippers and a pink candlewick dressing-gown. An ambulance had been sent to bring her for this out-patients appointment. She looked very, very old, a fixed crooked smile on her face, no teeth, hands almost immobile with swollen joints. Her daughter was in her sixties, and quite spry, though dreadfully tense and neurotic-looking.

It took a long time for Dr Silver to get the whole story. He started by approaching the mother. The GP's note was so short as to be almost non-existent. It mentioned bad ulcers on the legs from severe burns, and diarrhoea.

'Can you walk, Mrs Brown?' he asked quite loudly, but didn't seem to engage her attention. The daughter was about to answer but the doctor held out his hand to silence her. 'CAN YOU WALK, MRS BROWN?'

'Walk? Walk?' she said, grinning back at him suddenly. 'Oh yes, I can walk, I've always walked. Not well,' and she nodded her head as if once she had started it going she wasn't going to be able to hold it still again.

'No doctor, she doesn't walk at all. I have to carry her. She won't even try,' the daughter said, but the mother wasn't listening. The mother, in the wheelchair looked much bigger than the thin anxious daughter; it was difficult to imagine her lifting the old woman.

'WHAT ELSE IS THE MATTER, MRS BROWN?' he bellowed at the old woman again. She smiled at him and seemed to shake her head in an almost apologetic manner. It was as if she was somewhere near understanding where she was and what was going on, but just couldn't quite break through some impenetrable barrier that had cut her off. She didn't look unhappy.

'I'M JUST GOING TO TALK TO YOUR DAUGHTER SO WE CAN GET EVERYTHING IN THE RIGHT ORDER, ALL RIGHT?' the doctor shouted politely, but Mrs Brown just smiled and nodded and started to suck her lips in, until her already-cavernous cheeks sunk right into her skull.

Mrs Brown's daughter was polite, and waited to be asked questions before volunteering information. It wasn't until towards the end of the interview that she suddenly held forth, thinking that the doctor had not understood at all the nature of the case. Her story came out in disjointed stops and starts.

'How long have you been worried about your mother?' he asked.

'Oh she's been like this for years. Mostly it's her bowels, everything runs out of her.'

'Has she had diarrhoea for long?'

'Yes, a good nine years now I'd say.'

'When you say nine years, how often a year do you mean?'

Well, I give her this medicine to constipate her, kaolin morphine I think it is. It binds her. Yesterday she was haemorrhaging a bit with it so I called the warden. I'd say she gets it quite a lot of days every month.'

'She's been here before, hasn't she, a week ago? She saw the gynaecologist?'

'It was about her waterworks. It just runs out of her. He sent her to you, see?'

'Yes, I'm sorry for that. She shouldn't have been sent to the gynaecologist at all. I don't know how that happened.'

'Well, she wets herself a lot, you see.'

'How long has she been doing that?'

'Over two years now.'

'Does she ever have her motions running away from her? Is she "doubly incontinent", as we call it?'

'Yes, often. I've got her living with me. The washing!'

'So she's had trouble holding her water for two years. Is that day and night? When does she wet herself?'

'Oh, sitting down or standing up, any time.'

'Bed wet every night?'

'Two or three times a week.'

'Very wet or just a bit?'

'Oh, very, very wet. Oh, it is wet, doctor.'

Dr Silver paused while he was taking some notes. The daughter shifted uncomfortably in her chair.

'Doctor, you see it's like this,' she said, clearing her throat, and her voice squeaking from nerves. Her fingers were twitching at the clasp of her handbag as if she was dying for a smoke. 'They wanted to put her away in South Ockenden where she was living. They were going to put her away, because she was in such a state, especially with her bowels. But the only place they'd take someone with her bowels was a mental home. They hadn't a proper place to put her, and I wasn't having her in a mental home. So I didn't know what to do. I thought if I brought her up here to live with me, I'd find her a place to go where I could be near, see?' She paused to see what impression she was making before going on, with very little encouragement from the doctor.

'I've only got a one-bedroomed flat and it's on the third floor. I can't take her out. She never goes out. She's been living with me two months now. I sleep on the sofa. I've got a disc myself, doctor, and I can't hardly lift her. I've phoned the GP. But he never came.'

'You mentioned a warden before?'

'They're old people's flats. I'm sixty-four myself so I qualified for one. We have a warden to keep an eye.' She said this with even more anxiety in her voice. She was scrutinizing the doctor's face hard. I guessed she was afraid that having revealed she was in an old people's flat would register in the doctor's mind that it was a perfectly suitable place to keep the old lady. She seemed already to suspect that the doctor was not going to take her mother in. Perhaps she had tried other places before.

'You ought to hear how old I am! You'd be surprised! Oh yes, surprised!' said the old lady suddenly breaking out of her silent nodding.

'YES, MRS BROWN, I KNOW YOU'RE VERY OLD!' Dr Silver shouted.

He thumbed through the file in front of him, apparently deep in thought.

'Has she given up the flat in South Ockenden?' he asked.

'Yes. I had to when I brought her up here.' Some of the muscles in his face seemed to tighten.

'She kept burning her legs. That's how she got these ulcerations,' the daughter said. 'She's burnt her legs sitting in front of the gas fire three times in five years. And the flat was in such a state. You've never seen the like. She was supposed to have a home help come in and clean, but no one ever came.'

'Has she improved at all since she's been with you?'

'No. I wouldn't say she has. It's the cleaning, doctor, that I can't manage. It'd be all right if it wasn't all the washing.'

'You could have the Incontinent Laundry Service do that for you.'

'But they don't collect often and I couldn't have that smelly washing lying around waiting. I wash it all myself in the bath.' She stopped a minute, looking down at her hands, which were twitching again. 'I get no help from anywhere. I'm a divorcee, you see. My daughter, she'll tell you, it's all too much for me.'

'Does your mother have any other children or relations?'

'No. I'm the only one.'

Dr Silver turned to the mother again and began to question her.

'MRS BROWN, DO YOU KNOW HOW OLD YOU ARE?'

'Eighty-six or eighty-seven?' she answered with a little thought.

'YOU'RE EIGHTY-FIVE. CAN YOU REMEMBER WHEN YOUR BIRTHDAY IS?'

'OH, er. Yes, yes. Saturday something.'

'WHAT YEAR IS IT?'

'Yes. Well. America. Was it now? 1995? No, I think ... 1951 it is.'

'IT'S 1975, Mrs Brown. WHEN WERE YOU BORN?'

'1892,' she answered without a moment's hesitation, but got it wrong.

Dr Silver told her daughter to take her to the next room to get her undressed for an examination.

When she was ready he went in and looked at her as she lay on the bed. She groaned and shouted out a loud, 'OOH!' when he moved her legs.

After he had finished examining her, he came back into his cell-like consulting room, closing the door behind him, and slowly, methodically washed his hands while he explained to me what he thought of the situation.

'I can see that if we do take her in we'll have a near-impossible job of getting the daughter to take her back ever again. I'm not altogether sympathetic with the daughter. She's given up her mother's flat. She's made her homeless. She appears to have refused a hospital place that was offered in South Ockenden. I wonder if it really was a mental hospital? The best I can do is to delay, hold her off for as long as possible. On the other hand, if we took the mother in at once today, as the daughter's obviously hoping, we'll get the daughter's good will on our side, and that's important. I'm thinking that we might do a deal with her as we do with many other patients' relatives. We'll take her in for six weeks, and then send her out for six weeks. That way you can give the relatives six weeks' rest, and not use up so much of a hospital bed. It's so important to stop the patient becoming institutionalized. Many patients are on a rota of six weeks in, six weeks out. Right now, though, I'm not sure the daughter would accept that.'

It hardly ever happens that confronted with Dr Silver and his team, a relative dares actually to refuse point blank to take their parent home. It is a very difficult thing for anyone to do. But there is always that possibility, and the person would be well within their rights; they could always dump the old parent and leave, if they dared.

The daughter wheeled her mother back into the room. The daughter seemed to have been desperately thinking over what else she could say.

'I'm up to here with it, doctor. It's all her water trouble and the bowels. It's her memory. She won't even try not to do it. I get no help, no laundry, no nothing. I tell you I'm on valium all the time.'

'Well, I want you to see the social worker. She'll come and visit you and see what can be done,' the doctor said. 'I would also like to see your mother in a week to do some more tests. I want a surgeon to do a test to see if there's anything the matter that might be causing the diarrhoea. Then, when we get the results and the reports, we can all sit down and decide what to do next.'

The daughter looked utterly crushed and close to tears. The last hope that he would admit her mother immediately was finally taken from her. The week ahead stretched out before her interminably.

'Something will have to be done,' she said with what little resolution she had left. 'The soiling is so difficult. She's so obstinate. She often won't even let me lift her when I try to get her to the toilet. She does it on the floor out of spite. She tells you she walks but that's a lie. My daughter'll tell you, our neighbours'll tell you. She won't walk at all. Oh, she's definitely deteriorated such a lot, doctor. And my children live so far. They're no help. They live in South Ockenden, miles away.' She was pleading.

'South Ockenden? Was your mother living near your children?'

She thought perhaps she had revealed something, but wasn't sure what. There was a pause as she tried to rouse some dignity and not to allow herself to plead. The mother was still grinning and nodding. She looked happy and benign. (But the doctor

254

admits that most geriatric patients are gentle and bidding with doctors and strangers, angels in hospital, but when they get home they can be obstinate, violent and abusive with their relatives.)

'What will happen then?' the daughter asked.

'She will have the tests and we'll see,' he said firmly.

Slowly, and with a terrible look of resignation, the daughter rose to her feet, picked up her handbag, and turned to wheel her mother out of the door. She managed a polite smile to Dr Silver, and said, 'Thank you,' though it wasn't clear what for.

Dr Silver said, when they had gone, that he would probably admit this woman, but the strain on the resources of his department with each new long-term admission meant that he had to try every other alternative first.

More patients were seen next, the first suffering the early stages of Parkinson's disease, the second with a weak heart, the others with vaguer complaints. They were all women patients that morning, hardly surprising since about seventy-five per cent of the geriatrics in the borough are women. 'Women live much longer,' explained Dr Silver. 'Men tend to die very quickly if their wives die first. They can't manage on their own. But women seem to survive all right when their husbands die.'

Sadly, time spent in a geriatric department dismisses some of the nicer myths about old age. There are not many happy old Darby and Joans living out the golden autumn of their lives together, supporting one another kindly as they hobble off into the sunset. Dreadful, harsh and degrading things happen to couples who have been happily married all their lives.

It is almost bound to happen that if both people live to a ripe old age, the faculties of one will deteriorate before the other. Senile dementia is a terrible, cruel complaint. Victims undergo a drastic change of character. The quietest, gentlest old person can become violent, obscene, spiteful and unbearable. He may suffer delusions, invent lies about their past life, use any weapon to hurt the person he has loved most – and these changes are more than most husbands or wives can bear. The whole of their previous life can appear to them in a new light. They find it difficult to believe that their spouse has undergone a complete change of character – they suspect that underneath a calm and happy exterior, for all those years these dreadful thoughts and hatreds have been festering – that their life before was a lie and a deception, and that this was the truth.

It happens far more often that women have to suffer seeing their husbands change like this, before their eyes. The burden of deciding to put away a husband or wife is far harder than for a child to relinquish a parent to care. Spouses will struggle on for a long time with a husband or wife who has become detestable and vile, as well as disabled and incontinent, while they themselves may be far from strong.

Mr Cohen was waiting outside to see Dr Silver. His wife had been Dr Silver's patient for many years, and the doctor knew the family well. The man was alone, having left his wife at home. He didn't have an appointment, but begged to be allowed to talk to the doctor. He had waited quietly, with his cap in his hand until all the other patients had been seen.

The Sister told Dr Silver that Mr Cohen was waiting to see him urgently about his wife. Dr Silver gave an almost imperceptible sigh. 'I'd rather not,' he said. He seemed to know what was going to be said. 'I saw him just a few days ago when his wife was discharged. Can anyone else see him?'

'The other doctors still have long queues,' the Sister said firmly. 'And he's insisting on seeing you.'

'Oh well, I suppose I shall have to. But I'd rather have put him off for the moment.'

Dr Silver glanced through Mrs Cohen's file which the Sister handed to him. He scarcely needed to refresh his memory on a case so familiar to him already.

Mr Cohen was shown in. He was a small muscular red-faced man, remarkably fit and springy on his toes. He sat down quickly opposite the doctor, and put his cap on his knees. He was nearly bald. He had a part-time job as a butcher: he did the job because he said he would go mad if he had to sit at home with his demented wife all day, so he couldn't look after her properly.

256

A district nurse came in every morning to help her get up.

A few years ago his wife had undergone a colostomy for cancer of the colon. She now had to have a colostomy bag attached to her stomach all the time. She was very demented, and often fell. She had just been discharged from the hospital having had a fractured hip mended.

'Doctor, I tell you,' he said, leaning across the table a little, 'I've had a bad time, a very bad time in the last four days since you sent her out of hospital. I can't leave her alone for a minute. I tell you she's fallen three or four times already since I've had her back. It was Monday, when I came back from the Synagogue, she had fallen again. And I couldn't get into the room for the smell. It was terrible. Her bag on the floor, diarrhoea everywhere. Then she went on the floor again.'

'The motions were loose? She really had diarrhoea?'

'Doctor, according to the mess I had to clear up you'd say she had diarrhoea.'

'I wish you had agreed to see the other doctor today. She is his patient at the moment while she is attending the day hospital.' An ambulance called three days a week to collect Mrs Cohen.

'It's you I have to talk to. It's you that makes the decisions,' Mr Cohen said obstinately. 'But I'll tell you something, she fell in the ward on Wednesday, didn't she? She got a terrible bad black eye. It was a disgrace to send her home in that condition. As you know, she's got a stroke in her right side.'

'You know Mr Cohen, that a black eye may not be serious at all, it can just look dreadful. You agreed that we'd try her on a six-week rota. We'd take her for six weeks to give you a rest, and then you'd take her back for six weeks. You really haven't given it a try.'

'I wish you'd see her, what she's like at home. You say she was walking in hospital, well she won't walk at all at home.'

'I'd rather the other doctor saw her in the day hospital. He knows your wife very well indeed.'

'Doctor,' he said earnestly, leaning harder on the table, 'day hospital isn't enough. Six weeks at home is too much.' He paused and twisted his cap. 'I'd like to put her somewhere she can be looked after all the time. I just can't do it all the time. If I even go out she screams at me and then she falls on purpose when I've gone. You can't stop watching her for a minute.'

'You're still working?'

'I've just had to retire now.'

'How old are you?'

'I'm seventy-seven. I've packed up the working now. Much as I want to be at home the monotony of things at home is beyond me. I have to stay there all the time in case she wants to go to the toilet. All day long she screams and shouts at me. It's DO THIS or DO THAT! I can't stand it.'

He stared hard at Dr Silver to see if he had made any impact. Dr Silver slowly turned his pen in his fingers and then looked up at Mr Cohen.

'Well,' he said with a sigh, 'you've only had her home for four days. She may settle down. I don't think you've really given it a fair trial. But I'll send the other doctor to come and see you both this week, and then we'll discuss what should be done. I really think you must give it a good trial.'

Mr Cohen took some hope from the tone of resignation he detected in Dr Silver's voice. He suspected, probably rightly, that in the end, Dr Silver would have to capitulate. But it was impossible to tell how soon that end would be achieved. Mr Cohen took up his cap and went out of the room with a smile and a small wave.

When he had gone Dr Silver explained something of his view of the Cohen case to the other doctor, who came in. 'Well, I know it sounds very hard, but I know this husband well. I just didn't want to fall in with all this so easily.' He paused. 'From the nursing point of view she is a terrible problem, a lot of work in a ward. While she was in hospital she was continent and she could walk, though not well. But I know him. He doesn't like the worry of looking after her, or the trouble. He's always been rather strange about it. He still likes to go out, even though when he gets back he finds she's

fallen over and can't get up. He's only had her back four days!
He paused. 'I suppose in the end we'll have to cave in. We can
make an appointment to see her in out-patients next week.
Meanwhile we'll get the social worker to make inquiries about
getting her into a Jewish home. That'll probably take time.
There's a long waiting list. Does that seem a practicable
solution to you?'

'Yes, I think so,' said the other doctor.

'We shall take her in, but for the time being remind him
that he agreed to the six weeks in, six weeks out.'

It was arranged that she would probably go to St Matthew's,
the long-stay geriatric hospital, if she was admitted. I said I
thought he had been hard on the old man. Dr Silver drew a
deep breath.

'My greatest responsibility is to my patient,' he said.
'Sometimes there is a conflict of interest between the patient
and the family. I also have to remember that my second
responsibility is to provide the best possible services for all the
old people in the borough, and the resources are limited. If
we take her in I am saying to Mr Cohen, all right, I will take
the whole responsibility off your shoulders, and instead of
you helping, I am having to get nurses, doctors and domestic
staff to do it for you, and there is a great shortage of staff.
Instead of sharing her hospital bed with someone else, by
doing a six-week rota, you will be depriving another family
of even their six weeks' rest. A GP may be able to take the
whole family more into consideration, as they are all his
patients, but I have to look after my patient and all my other
patients.' In fact Mrs Cohen was admitted shortly afterwards,
and she died a few months later.

The out-patient clinic was over. The Sister came in and sat
down with Dr Silver, over a cup of coffee. She read out the list
of patients who had failed to turn up. Each of them had been
carefully checked on. 'Mrs Hoxton, refused to come when the
ambulance called. Mrs Gradey refused. Mrs O'Malley refused.
Mrs Goodbody said she wasn't well enough today. Mr Frost
called and made a new appointment. Oh yes, Mrs Sullivan

says she won't come again, but she's said that often before.'

The corridor was empty when we came out. There was a smell of lunch in the air and we went into the canteen.

As we ate I tried to get Dr Silver to talk about himself, but he was a quiet and reticent man. He was more humble about himself and his work than any other doctor I had met in the hospital. Several people in other departments had spoken of him with great admiration for his dedication. He described his career briefly, 'I had completed my training as a chest specialist, but the great decline in TB meant it was a narrowing field with few vacant posts. Like many other doctors at that time who found the delay before getting a consultant post interminable, I looked abroad, including Canada which I visited on a scholarship. The chance of starting as a geriatrician in this district, which I knew well, came up. Not very many geriatricians had been appointed. It was a new subject and I took the chance.'

Geriatrics is known as the Cinderella of medicine, and I could see why. There is not much glory to be earned for the geriatrician, just the quiet knowledge that he is alleviating suffering as best he can. Dr Silver is unlikely to make medical history in a big way. Though he speaks with optimism himself when he says, 'Research in geriatrics has been specially concerned with the extent of disease, often unrecognized among the elderly and how this can be dealt with. Geriatric departments themselves are experiments and operational research is important in dealing with the difficult problems of great and increasing numbers of old people, especially the very old. When such people are in difficulties there are very often medical causes. Few resources, old hospital buildings and inadequate staffing are other great problems and it is an enormous struggle to do things in the best way. How they are done is therefore very important. Until very recently research has had very little support from university departments. Problems like incontinence are so huge and overpowering and so unattractive that they have not received much sustained attention. More purely medical matters are now being studied. For example, the liability to fracture in elderly people due to Vitamin D deficiency. The opportunities for research are enormous and should lead to practical results.'

Yet it is hard to think that Mr West, the great joint replacement pioneer surgeon is even in the same profession as Dr Silver, not because his skills are greater but just so different. Dr Silver does have one thing named after him, a test called the Silver Test to see how confused or demented an elderly patient is. It is a series of questions checking old people's memory, orientation, speech, vision, manual dexterity, ability to read, etc.

In the out-patients' clinic I had been struck by his firmness with relatives of the old. I asked him about it, and he had a very clear and straightforward moral view. First of all, he said, he had been appalled when he came to the hospital to find so many patients kept in bed all day. His predecessor at the hospital, Lord Amulree, a pioneer geriatrician, had started the process of getting them up, and he continued it. He realized that all the people there would be better off at home if at all possible, alone if necessary, with relations, or if unavoidable, in an old people's home. 'It was my first aim to get as many of them out of here as I could, and to stop too many becoming institutionalized like them,' He said quite often people were still trying to hive off their responsibilities to their relatives. 'The State cannot possibly shoulder the whole burden, and even if it could, I do not see why it should,' he said.

After lunch Dr Silver was going on a ward round back at Mile End Hospital, his headquarters, and the main part of his department. Here were the most hopeful cases, and the atmosphere was more like that of The London Hospital than any of the other parts of Dr Silver's domain.

Mercer Ward is where patients are put who require assessment. With luck most of them will be returned soon to the outside world. They may have had fractures, or almost any other kind of ailment, but these are the ones who have been admitted as regular routine hospital cases with specific complaints. It is an acute, not a chronic ward. Here Violet Miller had been brought, as a regular emergency, until her long-term condition could be determined. These patients would either be released, sent to the rehabilitation ward on the top floor if they were going home or to an old people's home, or else sent on to St Matthew's for long-term care, or St Clement's if they turned out to be suffering from senile dementia.

It was the best and liveliest part of the geriatric department. Dr Silver had little trouble getting doctors and nurses to work here, as many of the patients were hardly distinguishable from the majority of those in general medical or surgical wards in the rest of the hospital. The ward is in a bright and airy modern block. It has small rooms with six beds each leading off a long wide corridor. Some of the rooms are for men, some for women, so that there is as little segregation as possible at meals and in the day room.

But there is no getting away from the fact that although it is thoroughly washed and cleaned every day, the place smells strongly of urine. It is distressing for visitors. Perhaps the patients don't notice it; the doctors and nurses don't seem to either.

Dr Silver arrived a little late and came hurrying down the corridor. Much of his life is spent bustling from one hospital to another spread out across the large borough.

The round began at the end of the ward, attended by the four doctors (they worked in pairs, taking half the patients each), the Staff Nurse, and two pupil nurses.

In the first bed of the first room was a tall old lady with cropped grey hair, lying on the counterpane, apparently asleep, her head cradled in her hands. As she lay there with her eyes shut she moaned and groaned and murmured to herself. Whatever was going on in her mind was sad and painful. One of the young doctors had her file and read out her case. 'Agnes James, eighty-four, deteriorating leg ulcers. Seems very confused, very difficult to understand anything she says. Her legs are too bad at the moment to walk.'

The Staff Nurse said, 'The legs are really dreadful. They smell terrible, and we keep trying to clean them up, but they aren't a lot better.' Dr Silver said she looked very dry. 'We're trying to make her drink, but she's hardly taking any.'

'What about the bacteriology?' he asked.

'We haven't had any results from the labs,' said the young doctor with a sigh. 'Their delays are getting worse and worse. We can't start her on antibiotics until we get a reading from the lab and she's in terrible pain. I've asked them to hurry, but they get angry with us.'

'The toes are gangrenous,' said Dr Silver as he gazed at the dreadful raw legs. The woman seemed quite unaware of the group round her bed. 'Is she a demented lady?' Dr Silver asked.

The others said they didn't really know, she was so confused.

'Put a nasal tube down her. We must hydrate her,' said Dr Silver and they passed on to the next case.

They came to an old lady with a grossly deformed leg from an operation to clear osteomyelitis as a child. The scar had become infected, as it frequently did. She was a bright and alert woman, the talker in the ward.

'When she came in she was terribly confused, but that's better now, isn't it?' said the nurse to the woman.

'Oh, I'm fine. Just want to get this healed and get back home,' she said. Patients didn't seem to mind being called 'confused'.

Sitting in a chair by the window was a fat old woman, asleep with a wide smile on her face.

'How are you today?' Dr Silver asked loudly.

She heard enough to wake up with a jump and say, 'Beg pardon?' still with a wide and slightly vacant smile.

'She's deaf as a post. You'll have to shout,' one of the doctors said.

'HOW ARE YOU?' Dr Silver bellowed.

'Thank you, yes, thank you doctor,' she said.

'HOW ARE YOU?'

'Oh better. I'm looking forward to going back to Donny-brook.' Donnybrook is one of the local old people's homes.

'Don't pick it!' The nurse said to her sharply, as the old

woman had nervously lifted her hand to pull at a piece of sticking plaster on her forehead.

'She's a bit slow, sleeps a lot, and we don't know why,' Dr Silver said thoughtfully. He got out a rubber hammer and rapped it hard a few times on her arm. She winced. The noise of the hammer on the bone was resonant.

'Go on then, why don't you all have a bash?' the old woman chuckled as the doctor continued the banging.

Dr Silver discussed the possibility of thyroid deficiency.

The young woman doctor assigned to this patient looked pleased. 'I like thyroid deficiency,' she said. 'They always make such a rapid improvement when you treat them.'

The same young woman doctor explained to me that this patient would probably be one of the healthier ones in a welfare home. 'In the old days, before Dr Silver came, the welfare homes would only take healthy old people. They aren't hospitals and only the matron is a trained nurse. But since Dr Silver's policy of trying to keep all the ones who can survive in the community, with relatives, or in their own flats, the only people to be sent to welfare homes are the ones too disabled to manage. The matrons of the homes hate this. They haven't got the staff or the facilities to deal with badly disabled people. They want nice clean sane old folk, the sort who have no reason for being there.'

Conversation with the next patient was as difficult. She too was quite deaf. She too had been asleep when the doctors approached.

'Are you better?' asked Dr Silver.

'Oh yes,' she said when she had finally understood the question. 'I can even tot along on me own a bit now.'

'How's the appetite?' She had been brought in with bad vitamin deficiency and appetite loss.

'I'm eating all right,' she said.

'What did you eat at home?'

'Oh nice meals, nice meals. I'd have milk, and some Oxo and half a slice. I like to drink a bit of that stuff that gets you on, too.'

'Lucozade?' Dr Silver was quick at interpreting old people's phrases.

'That's the one. I want to go home now. I know exactly what to eat now. It won't happen again.'

'Can you remember what you had for Christmas lunch?'

She thought for a long time. 'No, I'm sorry doctor, I can't, to be honest,' she said.

'Have they been talking to you here about what you should eat?'

'Well, they've been giving it me!' Everyone laughed. Then the doctor tested her eyes, which were very bad. He held up three fingers and asked her how many there were. She wasn't sure.

'Can you read very big print?'

'Oh no. Not at all.'

'Have you ever been able to read?'

'I should think so!'

'Can you see what this picture is?' he asked holding up a magazine with a girl on the front.

'Is it a dog?' she asked tentatively. He patted her hand warmly. He seemed more relaxed and kindly with old people than with anyone else, and they appeared to sense it.

Sitting by the last bed in the ward was a cross old lady who caused a lot of trouble to the nurses, and was not liked. She had several relatively minor ailments, but had really been taken in so that her son, with whom she lived, could go on holiday. These social admissions were frequent and are generously offered by the hospital to make life for relatives as easy as possible.

She was demented, had a terrible bunion, great difficulty in walking, was very deaf and suffered from arthritis. She lived with her son, but once she was admitted he had told the hospital firmly that he didn't want her back. She was supposed to attend the day centre three days a week to help take pressure off the family, but she had refused. She had refused to have meals on wheels, out of obstinacy, and had made life so bad for the home help that the home help had refused to go in any more. Alone in the house while her son was at work she had twice set her hair on fire with the gas cooker. She had almost fallen off a balcony, and kept trying to go out alone and had fallen on the outside concrete steps.

'She's a terror, even while she's here,' the Staff Nurse said, while they were out of her hearing, which wasn't very far. 'Her son says she's even worse at home. She tells us off all the time. She's always the one that has to be washed and dressed first. She has to have her meals first.'

'Does she accept the day hospital now?' Dr Silver asked.

'Yes, but she'll probably refuse to go again as soon as she gets home,' the nurse said.

'I think it may be hard to get the son to take her back. That's always the risk when we take people in for these social admissions. It's often much harder to get people to take them back again afterwards,' said Dr Silver sadly.

'The son says she keeps them awake all night and she doesn't sleep. She won't take sleeping tablets. She screams out in the middle of the night several times, and they think she's fallen out of bed, but when they get into her room she just wants to know what time it is,' said the nurse, who seemed to sympathize with the woman's son.

The doctor asked the woman to show him how well she could walk. Like many of the patients on the ward she walked slowly with a metal frame for support. She looked mild and friendly. 'I'm good at it now, aren't I?' she said. She didn't look like a tyrant.

The doctor examined her feet.

'She needs a chiropodist. Can you arrange that, nurse?'

'We haven't got one any more, I'm afraid.'

'Not at all? Nowhere in the whole hospital?'

'The lady who used to come has part-retired now. All she does is one afternoon at Whitechapel. She won't come to Mile End. She won't do geriatrics any more.'

'But it must be possible to get one from somewhere?'

'There just aren't any. No one wants to train for chiropody any more. They aren't paid well. We've tried all over the place,' one of the young doctors said.

'Well, I don't see how any of us can try our hands at it, do you?'

The doctors laughed and shook their heads.

The next room was all men. In the first bed was a small sad old man called George Hammond. He was lying on his bed with his dressing-gown and slippers on, doing nothing. Before going into the room one of the doctors summed up his case. He was a social admission. His wife was quite seriously ill and he had been taken in because his children refused to look after him. He was quite demented, and described as an 'ex-alcoholic' (presumably because no one could go on being an alcoholic in hospital). His wife had said firmly that she didn't want him back when she came out of hospital. She wanted him put away in a welfare home, as he beat her up all the time. The children said they wanted nothing to do with him. Here was a case not of a sweet old man turned senile and nasty, but of a nasty man who had bullied and battered his family all their lives, and now at last they had the chance to get rid of him. 'But since he came in, he suddenly developed bad oedema of one leg,' the doctor continued. They examined his leg, which was painful.

Dr Silver wondered what should be done with him. He thought the old man would probably do well in a welfare home, since he was the nicest, gentlest person in hospital with the nurses, whatever he was like at home – but he was reluctant to send him there until it was absolutely necessary. 'A welfare home is so drastic. Once you go in you're really there for ever. If we put him in a long-stay bed at St Andrew's Hospital, the family might change their minds. I don't know if his wife is really in a condition to make decisions.'

In the next bed was a man with grey skin and a deeply sunken face, from which a long nose protruded. He had lung cancer. 'Apart from tiredness and wheezing a lot, he seems to be pretty symptomless,' a doctor explained. The nurses liked him as he was friendly and quite talkative. He lived with his sister who wanted him back. The doctors were waiting for the results of tests which would tell them more or less how long he would live. If he had a reasonable life expectancy, they would release him at once, but it might be that he would die quickly, and they didn't want to cause his sister unnecessary suffering. X-rays showed that some of his ribs had been eaten away.

'The only thing about him,' the nurse said, 'is that he has trouble with buttons. He's obsessed with them. He eats them all off his pyjamas and trousers. He just pulls them off and swallows them down. Otherwise he's quite all right.'

When he walked down the corridor you could hear him coming from the far end. He walked fast, shuffling his big slippers along with great speed and dexterity, but his breathing made a dreadful noise, with chokes and squeaks, like a sick steam train.

The last two patients were the most ill in the ward. They were each kept in single rooms.

The first of these, Mrs Semple, was lying awake in a bed, with two cot sides attached to it to stop her falling out. She had a drip at the head of the bed, and a bag collecting urine from a catheter tube at the side. Her arms were bandaged to the side of the bed to stop her pulling out the drip. She had pneumonia, and had recently developed an obstruction of the bowel. Her abdomen was grossly distended.

'She's very distended,' the nurse said. 'She says she's had a baby. She went on saying that until we agreed. She talks to the baby all the time and calls it Jane. It seems to make her happy though.'

The nurses had eventually given her a doll – Dr Silver hated this, though admitted that it seemed to make the woman buoyantly happy.

Mrs Semple tried to tell the doctors about her 'baby', but had trouble in talking. They prodded her abdomen, and were not happy about her condition.

'I think she's definitely going to have to stay in hospital,' Dr Silver said. He had been wanting to move her soon. He was beginning to wonder if she'd make it.

'We've been trying to arrange a place at St Matthew's, but

the family were horrified when we said she was going there. They said they'd never let her go there,' said a doctor.

'What are their objections?' Dr Silver asked, a little huffily.

'I think some neighbours of theirs said their grandmother had been left in there for years and they said it was a terrible old work-house. They warned her family against it.'

'These stories always get around,' Dr Silver said with a sigh. 'I wonder how long ago these neighbours are talking about? I don't suppose they've seen the place for years. We could arrange for the relatives to come and look round and perhaps they'd feel better about it then.'

The woman was dandling the doll on her knee and cooing to it. With her arms strapped to the cot sides she couldn't move much, but she seemed unaware of her captivity. The drip bottle shook a little as she rocked herself from side to side, and she hummed through her thin in-growing lips.

Violet Miller was in the next-door room, and she was the last call of the round. Everyone crowded into the small space and gathered round her bed. To me, she looked just the same, quite unchanged. She lay on her side, her face cradled in one hand. Her cheeks still looked pink and round. On closer inspection the becoming pink was from small broken blood vessels near the skin, and perhaps they keep their colour whatever the person's state of health.

We stood and looked at her for a moment before anyone said anything. To me she still looked pleasantly asleep, as if she might sit up and smile. But Dr Silver opened his file of medical notes, and after reading them for a moment or two, he shouted, making us jump, 'Violet, Violet!' If you stare at something long enough it's easy to believe it moved. I thought I could detect a flicker, just the faintest movement, a tiny sign of some hearing, some understanding. He tried again, 'Violet, wake up Violet!' he called again. Again I thought for a moment I saw half a twitch, but perhaps it was just the late afternoon sun reflecting on her face from the metal bed rails.

'Nothing,' said Dr Silver. He read through her notes again,

while the rest of us gazed at her. There was something about that peaceful sleeping face that held the eye.

Then he said that he had almost completely discounted their first diagnosis. If she had taken an overdose of anti-depressants the effects would have started to wear off by now. That, he was now almost certain, was not the explanation. He read out the result of yesterday's EEG tests. (They test the state of the brain.) The tests showed, he said, that the brain was scarcely functioning at all. 'I think we can safely say that this is a cerebrovascular disease,' he said. She had suffered a massive stroke. There was almost no brain left, she was almost dead already. She was a breathing replica of a human being, nothing more.

Dr Silver rolled the bed clothes off her gently. With the end of a small rubber hammer he tested the soles of her feet for reflexes, and was not pleased with the result, as he shook his head. I noticed her teeth were still sitting in their mug on the sink, and that there was still nothing personal in the room, not a bottle of orange juice, not a grape or a flower, not a get-well card, a dressing-gown, a pair of slippers, not a box of Kleenex, a copy of Woman's Own, not one single object of her own.

When he had finished his brief examination of her, one of the young doctors, whose patient she was, said, clearing his throat nervously, as if anxious not to appear presumptuous in pointing out something Dr Silver might have missed, 'She seems to be getting a little wheezy,' and coughed again.

Dr Silver raised his head from scribbling notes in her file, and he fixed the young man with a firm look. 'Well,' he said slowly, 'we won't give her antibiotics, I think.' The young man nodded his head in vigorous agreement, to show that he in no way disagreed with the patient's treatment. He realized, almost as soon as he said it, that Dr Silver had not by any means missed out these early symptoms of the first stages of pneumonia. He had simply preferred not to mention it. The young man felt foolish and blushed. Tact should have made him hold his tongue, let them all make a mutual, but silent agreement. If she had pneumonia, this poor vegetable should be allowed to die in peace.

They moved quickly out of the little room, trying to look as if nothing had been made in the way of a decision, though it had.

Apart from some office work, it was the end of Dr Silver's day. We sat down for a while in the conference room to drink some tea. The slanting sinking sun was catching the shine on some singularly unattractive photographs of geriatric devices – lavatory seats, bath rails, and tray slings.

Naturally Dr Silver did not like to talk about the possibility of shortening the more miserable lives of some of his patients. 'How could I do that?' he asked. 'What sort of unit could I run, what sort of practice could anyone run if they went about killing their patients?'

'But what is the purpose of medicine,' I asked, 'if not to relieve suffering?'

'How could I kill people?' he said. 'I couldn't, and wouldn't if I could.'

I asked him how he anticipated his own old age.

'With horror,' he said straight away. 'Of course I have no idea what the odds are of dying suddenly and quickly while in reasonably good health, against dying slowly and uncomfortably after a host of diseases. We don't collect those statistics.'

'What about death?'

'You or I would find it difficult to cope with the near-certainty that we should be dead within five years – a prospect squarely faced by anyone of eighty. Yet somehow I don't think they see it the same way. There is a slowing down, an acceptance, and we must hope for that.'

The 'Happy Death' was a very real concept to him. When I visited St Matthew's, the old work-house, it became very real to me too. I felt that Violet Miller was perhaps a lucky woman, and I was glad she would never wake up to find herself there.

St Matthew's Hospital is a sad place. It is hard to describe the grimness of it without appearing to blame someone – yet there is really nowhere to place the blame.

Although the hospital itself is understaffed, smelly and poverty stricken, in the middle of an especially grim part, on the Hackney border, it is the 180 patients themselves that make the place so deeply depressing. Numb and blank, they sit all day in their day rooms at the end of the wards, an ineradicable smell of urine, some of them gabbling to themselves, many mercifully asleep, with their toothless mouths agape. The sun tracking slowly across the room from one wall to the other provides the only change. They don't talk to one another. They don't appear to talk to visitors when they come. Visitors tend to come in pairs, and talk to one another.

Since his arrival Dr Silver had tried as hard as possible to stop St Matthew's looking like the work-house it began life as. The huge old wards with great metal cots close together have been modernized. The cast-iron supports have been removed from the ceilings, and the wards sectioned off in a more humane way. All the patients who are not seriously ill are got out of bed every day, into the day room at the end of the ward. Bright curtains have been put up. The entrance to the building has been modernized – instead of two great port-cullis gates looking like a prison there is a sort of plastic portico, looking like a cinema.

But there is something about the basic structure of the place that is quite unalterable. It was built for brutally utilitarian purposes. Half the corridors are subterranean and lined with fat lagged central heating pipes. As you enter the building, to get to the wards or the administration department you have to pass the strong-smelling kitchens, down in an underground passage, and up some stairs to an area that looks like a roof top, with curious glass sky-lights protruding from the ground. This dark walled yard has been given a facelift by the incongruous inclusion of a few little round tables and some furled stripey sun umbrellas.

One patient at the hospital had been born at St Matthew's,

when it was a work-house. I doubt whether the facelift fooled her much.

St Matthew's has more trouble recruiting staff than any of the other hospitals in the geriatric department. You could tell that with just a glance round the wards. All the nurses were wearing different uniforms – a sign that they were agency nurses. Some nurses were just passing through, some of the agency nurses had been there for a year or two. If agencies were closed down, this hospital would cease to function at all. There was a high proportion of coloured nurses. All the doctors there were Indian.

Dr Silver spent Fridays at St Matthew's. He started with a case conference in each ward. A motley group of nurses gathered round the desk in the first ward. The most senior nurse in charge of the ward was only a temporary and had been in the place a short day and a half. The two doctors were both women and both Indian. One of them, Dr Jena, had been at the hospital for some time and knew the patients well. The other was a locum standing in for a doctor who was on holiday. Dr Silver had not met the locum before and he introduced himself politely. It became immediately evident that she could not speak a word of English, and did not understand anything that was being said to her. Dr Jena kindly tried to prompt her, but to no avail. Dr Silver took this with polite and calm resignation. It was the sort of thing he often had to contend with at St Matthew's.

The catalogue of ailments was not so different from those in the ward at Mile End, but the patients were just in a worse state, and each had a longer list of complaints attached to her name.

Dr Jena went through all of the patients. It was a long, long list. When they came to an end Dr Silver asked,

'There's a cremation form on my desk for a Mrs Smith. Who is she?'

'She died two days ago. Broncho-pneumonia.'

'Did I know her?'

'I think you saw her once, bad arthritis and only one eye.'

'Oh yes. I think I remember.'

Cremation forms have by law to be signed by two doctors, verifying the cause of death and swearing that they know of no reason why the death should be regarded as suspicious. The second doctor need not have known the patient in life.

In one corner of the hospital is the day centre – the only reasonably cheerful part of St Matthew's. Here disabled old people are brought in ambulances, and some fit old people come in for a cheap hot lunch.

Lunch was being served by orderlies from a large trolley on wheels. Two ambulance drivers would bring patients in intermittently, wheeling them across the great hall at top speed, laughing and spinning them around, in what looked like an undignified and frightening fashion. The occupational therapist, however, was praising the drivers, saying how lucky they were to have found two volunteers prepared to do the job every day, rather than having to rely on a pool. These drivers knew all the patients and their foibles, and were adored by them. When they had recently gone on holiday, some of the old people had refused to be taken out by the relief drivers.

At some tables there were quite fit-looking people, chatting away to each other; at others were wheelchair occupants scarcely able to feed themselves. One of these carried a doll in her wheelchair which she sometimes pretended to feed. Her only conversation was about her 'baby'. Dr Silver said again he didn't really like to see this lady with her doll, but it seemed to make her happy, so he thought perhaps he was wrong to stand too much on human dignity.

Various activities were arranged each day at the centre – painting, singing, drama. The only odd thing about these activities is that they were called 'painting therapy', 'singing therapy', 'drama therapy'.

When Dr Jena had finished the tour of all the cases on her list, Dr Silver had time to pause a moment and talk about staffing problems at St Matthew's.

'A doctor, you see, trained in this country would not take this job as it now is. He would have a choice of other jobs which would suit him better. Some overseas doctors have come over here who were not very well qualified and did not speak good English. St Matthew's does give them a chance to settle and get used to the country. Sometimes they have particular personal reasons for coming here. In the past they all came for post-graduate training and returned home but now they have come because they want to settle, and some are refugees. They just come for a higher standard of living in this country, as they see it, to better themselves. We have had many very good doctors from overseas. Yes I do feel badly about our National Health draining away doctors from underdeveloped countries, but there's nothing we can do about it really, if they are determined to leave. Yes, I know that some of them are of very low standard, like this locum who can't speak English. She is at least a pair of eyes. She is much better than nothing, I can assure you, and nothing is the only alternative.'

One of the most poignant incidents I witnessed in the geriatric department concerned an ex-nurse. She was old and blind, foul tempered, and the worst patient by far in the rehabilitation unit. As I watched her, and the exasperation she caused those looking after her, I couldn't help asking a nurse there whether she didn't ever get overwhelmed with fears for her own old age.

'Oh God,' said the nurse, a pleasant middle-aged woman, 'you can't help thinking about it on your bad days. Yes, this patient, this ex-nurse I suppose is especially hard for us to deal with. Dear God, I pray it'll never be me!'

In a wheelchair at a table sat the blind old nurse, hair scraped back in a bun. She was hunched over her food. She was waiting for 'Part III', an old people's home, as soon as a place could be found. Not surprisingly they were having some difficulty in getting her accepted. She was methodically picking up pieces of tinned peaches with her fingers, putting them onto her spoon, and the spoon into her mouth. 'Stop talking, be quiet! You make too much noise!' she kept loudly saying from time to time to the absolutely silent old lady sitting inoffensively opposite her.

When they had all finished eating an orderly came and cleared away the plates. This disturbed the old lady in the wheelchair 'Where's my plate? Nurse! Where's my plate?' The orderly explained to her that she had finished and the plate had been taken away.

'Don't rush me! I had some fruit left on it. You took it away!' she said angrily.

'No dear,' said the orderly. 'You did very well and it was all finished.'

Dr Silver was looking through the old nurse's notes, with the ward Sister looking over his shoulder. At some point in one of the nurse's stays in another hospital someone had written down, 'This woman is a weary cross to bear for all who come in contact with her.' Dr Silver said regretfully that she was indeed troublesome, bossy, and unpopular.

'She was a nurse, an SRN in her day. I have a sort of feeling she must always have been a tyrant,' said Dr Silver.

The nurses hated her, though they were remarkably tolerant.

'What I can't stand about her,' said one nurse, 'is just because she was a nurse she thinks she knows it all. We can't tell her anything. She shouts that nurses and doctors have no right to make her do things. She'll never have an enema, for instance. Oh, she knows all the ropes.'

The old lady had been wheeled away from the table to a place beside the wall. 'I really don't know what we can do with her. She won't go to sing-songs, or play games. She just wages war. She drove them mad at St Andrew's. It'll be hard to find a place that will take her.'

'Does she have visitors?' Dr Silver asked.

'She has these Church people who have known her for years. They say she's always been this way, ungrateful and ordering them about,' said the Sister.

The woman called for a nurse to pick something up for her. The nurse obliged, then went to see another patient.

'Nurse!' she shouted again. The nurse was busy, and so were the others, so no attention was paid to her. She kept shouting 'Nurse! Nurse! Nothing will they do, this lazy good for nothing lot! Will nobody do anything? What ever has gone wrong with this ward? Are you all gone blind? Are you all gone deaf?'

Dr Silver said to the Sister, 'Perhaps she'd be happier with other nurses. Do you think we have a chance of getting her into a nurses' retirement home?' Sister didn't know but said she would try to find out.

As we left the ward the old nurse was shouting out like an aged war-horse still commanding her student nurses, 'This ward is a disgrace! An outrage! Where on earth do you think you nurses are? Nurse? Have you all gone stark mad, you insolent baggages? Mad? Are you all mad?'

The next day I saw Violet Miller in the morning, and she looked different – smaller, more hunched, and she wheezed heavily. A day later she died, peacefully, without moving a limb, without having given any sign of life, except in the loudness and heaviness of her breath. Her room was empty when I next passed it by – but it seemed to me as I looked through the open door that it didn't look much emptier than when she had lain there. She had never occupied it at all. She had never been in hospital. They hadn't been able to do anything to her there – either good or bad.

The nurse on duty in the office said, of course, that it was a blessing, and I agreed. They had many such blessings a year in the geriatric unit, but some were later in coming than others. Some came after five or more years in the misery of St Matthew's. Violet Miller's son said it was a blessing, so did Dr Silver. A chirpy young student nurse with platinum hair said it was a shame, such a lovely old lady. A Portuguese orderly swabbing the floor of the empty room crossed herself and murmured. The old man with lung cancer and a taste for buttons came belting down the corridor, nodded at the room, and shouted, 'She's a goner!' laughing at the top of his voice.

There is a corner of the main hospital at Whitechapel, a small screened-off piece of the admissions office called colloquially 'Dead Man's Corner'. The cotton screen doesn't keep out the bustle of coming and going in the office. On a desk is a great tome, the register of deaths, each death entered by hand in ink, signed by the doctor, and cause of death registered beside the name.

The dead person's possessions are brought here, waiting to be collected. There was an old violin under the table, willed by a dead patient to a man in Tasmania who never arrived to collect it. In Whitechapel there was an average of three deaths a day.

Outside the screen three young Turkish people were arguing in bad English with a stiff receptionist. All were elegantly dressed and good looking. They were quarrelling about the hospital's arrangements for burying their grandfather who had just died. 'I'm sorry,' said the receptionist, 'but we only provide one car. This is a hospital funeral, you know. If you want another car you must pay for it yourselves.'

The young man explained that they were all on social security and couldn't afford to. 'It doesn't show any respect!' one of the girls almost shouted. 'The relatives must follow the body from the hospital.'

'I'm afraid you'll have to make your own arrangements for getting to the funeral,' said the receptionist, losing her temper. 'You will just have to find the money to hire a car, or meet the funeral at the cemetery gates.'

'We know hospital funerals!' said the young man, almost spitting through his teeth. 'Cheap!'

'Listen, the hospital is very generous. A funeral costs us £45 and the death grant we get from the state is only £30.'

'Short service, cheap funeral!' said the other girl, and they all got up and stamped out.

The receptionist blew her top. 'What are they doing on social security anyhow, I'd like to know!'

An old man came in and was quietly waiting. He came up to the desk and gave his name. He explained that he had come for his wife's possessions. The receptionist went to ask whether anyone had some property for Mr Davis whose wife had died on Tuesday, in Turner Ward. The man stood patiently and looked at his shoes. He smiled shyly at some other people waiting near by.

The woman came back with a battered suitcase and two half-torn carrier bags. He took them. 'Would you please check carefully that everything is there, Mr Davis?' she said kindly. 'I'll just go and fetch the watch from the safe.' He looked through the bags. Everything was there – old worn slippers, some magazines, even a half-finished bottle of lemon barley water. She came back with the watch and as he put his hand out to take it, one of the carrier bags ripped and spilled the contents onto the floor. Several people scrambled to help him pick them up. 'Would you like a better bag, Mr Davies?' she asked.

He looked confused and said, 'No, I can manage.' He turned towards the door, but then turned back to her. 'I'd just like to say that I'm very grateful indeed for everything, very grateful,' he said. He put down a bag and held out his hand to shake hers. Then he went for the door. He was just going through it when the bag broke again, and again a hair brush, a pair of scissors and the slippers fell out. They found him another bag and helped him out of the room and down the corridor to the exit.